GOOD-BYE TO BAD BACKS

FOREWORD BY
Richard M. Bachrach, D.O.

PHOTOGRAPHS BY
John Vidol

LINE DRAWINGS BY
David Chevtaikin

Good-bye to Bad Backs

Stretching and Strengthening Exercises for Alignment and Freedom from Lower Back Pain

Second Edition

JUDITH SCOTT

A Dance Horizons Book

Princeton Book Company, Publishers
Pennington, NJ

To
My mother, Evelyn
My family and friends
and
All my students
Past, present, and to come.

You inspire me.

Photographs on page 20 are reprinted from Arthur A. Michele, *Iliopsoas*, 1962. Courtesy of Charles C. Thomas, Publisher, Springfield, Illinois.

A Dance Horizons Book
Princeton Book Company, Publishers
P.O. Box 57
Pennington, NJ 08534

Library of Congress Cataloging-in-Publication Data

Scott, Judith, 1937–
    Good-bye to bad backs : Stretching and strengthening exercises for alignment and freedom from lower back pain / Judith Scott.—2nd ed.
        p.   cm.
    "A Dance Horizons book."
    Includes bibliographical references and index.
        ISBN 0-87127-186-9
    1. Backache—Exercise therapy. I. Title.
RD768.S334   1992
617.5'64062—dc20   92-34672

Acknowledgments

As a choreographer and a teacher, I am accustomed to channeling my creative energies through the direction of people performing movement. Sitting still to write a book was a new creative experience for me. And I had to do it alone, or so I thought. Then I began thinking about all the people who were contributing their time, effort, and energy into making my idea become a reality.

My thanks to Dr. Hugo Keim for reviewing the book; to Dr. Ellen Manos for her critical comments on the chapter pertaining to pregnancy; and to my special friend, Dr. Norton Flanagan, for his comments and continued support during this project. And most especially I want to thank Gus Giordano for being my "guiding star."

Thanks to John Vidol for his photographs and David Chevtaikin for his illustrations; to my models George Buxton, Linda Conte, Meg Cox, Tina Glavan, and Susan Mayberger.

I am sincerely grateful for the helpful suggestions that have been expressed by the many readers of the first edition. I have tried to incorporate as many of their ideas as possible.

And, finally, my thanks to all the wonderful people who have been, are, or will be my students. Your questions have taught me that the best way to learn something is to try to teach it. This book is our collaboration in our quest for a healthier body.

Contents

Foreword

Judith Scott and I met for the first time in 1967 when she came to my office, her back a source of chronic pain. Her problems were resistant to my ministrations largely because of my own (at the time) tunnel-visioned approach to both diagnosis and treatment. Then, as now, there was a plethora of madly divergent concepts as to the causes, natural history, management, and prevention of back pain.

The greater mass of conventional medical and surgical wisdom at the time indicted the intervertebral disk (ruptured, bulging, and so on) as the villain. Those of us practicing manual or manipulative medicine considered vertebral malalignment, displacement or restricted motion to be the ultimate cause. Some of the more farsighted of my colleagues recognized the primacy of the involvement of muscles and ligaments and the interrelationship of psyche and soma. But each school tended to see things in the narrower context of its own area of expertise, and even to try to fit diagnosis and treatment into a preconceived system.

The biggest hurdle in the treatment of back pain is the determination of an accurate functional diagnosis. Thus, if the physician was of the "disk-is-everything school," those patients with disk disease would respond; however, when the disk was not the source, treatment would be unsuccessful and the patient would look elsewhere for relief. Likewise, we "bone-crackers" (as the medical establishment condescendingly referred to us) were at a loss applying our concepts to most cases of intervertebral disk herniation. Yet all of us had some degree of success treating most of our patients, strongly suggesting either that everyone got better, regardless (or in spite) of treatment or that there was some degree of merit to all of our approaches. The next logical extrapolation was that perhaps there were no essential differences between schools and that there is some sort of etiological continuum to the back pain story.

Was it possible that the classic herniated disk represented an advanced stage in the progression of the back pain syndrome? I believe this to be true in the great majority of recurrent lower back pain problems. Poor posture, associated with tightness and weakness (insufficiency) of the psoas, weak abdominal muscles, tight hamstrings, sedentary life-style, stress reaction and depression all combine to compress the spine and its interspacing cushions, the intervertebral disks. With disk compression and deformation there are disturbances in the biomechanical relationships of the small joints connecting the vertebrae, resulting ultimately in spinal arthritis.

The key, then, to management of lower back pain is prevention. In her book, *Good-bye to Bad Backs*, Judith Scott gives to the reader, for the first time, the tools to interrupt this process before it evolves into disk herniation (necessitating prolonged rest, extensive and costly treatment and/or expensive and possibly disabling surgery) or to irreversible and incapacitating spinal arthritis.

Judith herself is the best testimonial to the effectiveness of her theories and methods. She is one of the most active, healthy and energetic people I know—she is a teacher, a writer, a personal trainer, and runs her studio in New York City. And, best of all, applying the methods Judith has outlined in this book, she has said good-bye to her own bad back!

DR. RICHARD M. BACHRACH

Preface to the Second Edition

Since the first edition of *Good-bye to Bad Backs* was released, my students, peers, and colleagues have requested a chapter for dancers. It is a source of great pleasure to know that reader interest in the first edition of *Good-bye to Bad Backs* has been great enough to warrant a second edition with a new chapter for dancers and athletes that includes specific stretches beneficial to them. Additional photographs have been provided to ensure reader understanding of the release activities. There have been minor revisions and I have corrected the text throughout to provide a more accurate second edition.

Proper body mechanics is increasingly being accepted among dancers and athletes as the first way to prevent injury. Because bodies of dancers and athletes are the only instrument they can "play" to achieve their desired end, they must keep their bodies functioning optimally. Therefore, dancers and athletes have become much more sophisticated in understanding the scientific ramifications of correct biomechanics. Concurrently, broader access to dance and sports medicine has educated many dancers and athletes to the importance of the work included in the following pages to prevent injury.

Introduction
The Secret of the Psoas

An estimated 80 percent of the general population in America will experience significant lower back pain during their lifetimes. Approximately 28 percent of the total industrial population of the United States will experience disabling lower back pain at some time,[1] and 8 percent of all working people will be sent home from work each year because of lower back pain.[2] In the United States, back pain is the most frequent cause of limited activity in patients over forty-five years of age.[3] The loss of both money and productivity due to low back pain is larger than that due to any other health problem except the common cold.

Lower back pain can result from many different causes: structural problems (congenital abnormalities, fractures, etc.); inflammatory diseases (rheumatoid arthritis, etc.); neoplastic disorders (primary and metastatic tumors, etc.); metabolic disorders (hyperparathyroidism, etc.); and referred pain. In the majority of cases, however, no systemic cause can be identified as the initiating factor of lower back pain, which often leads to a diagnosis of muscle sprain or strain or of idiopathic (of no known cause) lower back pain. Most people with back pain can be reassured that no major disorder is causing it and that the pain can be relieved without surgery.

Recent scientific evidence indicates that recurring back pain

**Results of PEPCO (Potomac Electric Power Company)
Study of 5,380 Employees**

	First Year	Second Year
Percent of decrease in number of patients with lower back pain	29	44
Percent of decrease in days lost	51	89
Percent of decrease in surgery for lower back pain	88	76
Cost of savings in time lost	$201,000	$302,000

can be reduced and possibly even eliminated with a program of exercise that includes regular stretching and strengthening. For example, in a study[4] at the Potomac Electric Power Company (PEPCO), 5,380 employees who complained of lower back pain between July 1981 and July 1983 were referred to a back clinic. Patients visited the rehabilitation program weekly or biweekly until they were ready to return to work. Over the two years of the program, there were substantial reductions in the number of patients treated, surgical procedures required, and days lost from work when compared with the prestudy years.

Despite this reassuring news, however, it is interesting to note that Arthur C. Klein and Dava Sobel, authors of *Backache Relief*,[5] reported that only 15 percent of physicians and 26 percent of other health-care practitioners list exercise as part of the rehabilitative process in treating back pain. Most specialists have little or no training at all in the study of back exercise. A study reported in the *Journal of Medical Education* in 1975 indicated that the typical medical student spent "an average of about four hours . . . studying the effects of exercise" on back pain. Based on the research conducted for their book, Klein and Sobel concluded that an individual exercise program is crucial to the recovery of anyone who is suffering from disabling back pain.

Back pain can result from many causes, but most often lower

back pain emanates from soft-tissue involvement of the muscles, tendons, and ligaments that accompany spinal injuries. Patients with herniated or "slipped" disks who attend the Comprehensive Pain and Rehabilitation Center in Miami are treated much the same as patients whose only apparent lower back problem is muscle spasm and tightness. Their rehabilitative program begins with stretching exercises followed by abdominal muscle strengtheners and instruction in proper body mechanics. *Good-Bye to Bad Backs* uses the same principles of stretching your psoas muscle and lower back, strengthening your abdominals, and improving your overall posture to help you say "bye-bye to bad backs and bulging bellies." This book shares with you the secret of the psoas.

THE SECRET OF THE PSOAS

We can all feel, by touching, the muscles that ache when we get up in the morning after a terrible night's sleep, the muscles that seem to "give out" in the middle of the workday when all we've been doing is sitting, the muscles that still hurt as we're watching the late night news and preparing for yet another terrible night's sleep, right? Wrong!

The culprit *isn't* touchable. It's buried deep within the body, where it supports some seven-eighths of the weight of the abdominal organs. This muscle group, known as the iliopsoas, or simply the psoas (pronounced *SO-as*), is indispensable to good health, yet most of us don't even know it's there, let alone how imperative it is to keep it in tip-top shape.

The psoas muscle has been a well-guarded secret. Twenty-five years have passed since orthopedic surgeon Arthur A. Michele, M.D., published the pioneering work *Iliopsoas* in which he set forth his theory that it is this muscle group that plays a central role in the treatment of lower back pain:

> I have in this work expounded my theory that practically all conditions . . . are attributable, in the main, to one basic lack in man, and that is his failure to elongate the Iliopsoas musculature to an extent commensurate with his anthropological progression towards the erect posture.

It is my firm belief that any and all defects of the spine and the hip joint structures should be evaluated in terms of disturbance of function of the Iliopsoas, a hitherto unrecognized prime mover, in the etiology of those defects.[6]

Although osteopathic physicians, orthopedists, physical therapists, coaches, and trainers have long recognized the importance of this major muscle group, the general public is virtually unaware of its existence.

WHAT IS THE PSOAS?

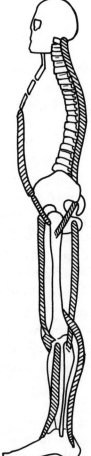

Whether you are standing still or in motion, your muscles must be constantly balancing all of your body segments or you would collapse in a heap on the floor. Because your body is flexible, the job of staying erect against the force of gravity makes far greater demands on certain muscle groups than on others. Those muscles responsible for holding the body upright are known as the postural muscles. When the pull of these muscles is evenly balanced, the body stands erect. The primary postural muscles involved in erect posture are the calf muscles (gastroc-soleus) and the iliopsoas in concert with the gluteus maximus. The secondary postural muscles include the abdominal muscles and the muscles supporting the spine (see Figure 1).

The iliopsoas muscle group consists of the psoas major, the psoas minor, and the iliacus (see Figure 2). The psoas major —the most important postural muscle of the group—arises from deep within the body, from the intervertebral disks between the lumbar vertebrae, which begin at the bottom of the rib cage and proceed down the lower back, and continues diagonally through the center of the torso and over the rim of the pelvis, where it attaches to the inside of the thigh bone (see Figure 3). We will refer to the iliopsoas muscle group simply as the psoas.

Because the psoas muscle extends through the center of the body, connecting the lower back to the front of the torso, where it helps to support seven-eighths of the abdominal contents, it is easy to understand its importance as a primary postural muscle.

Figure 1.
The postural muscles.

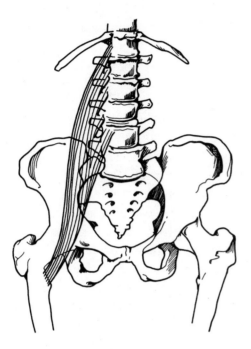

Figure 2. The iliopsoas muscle group.

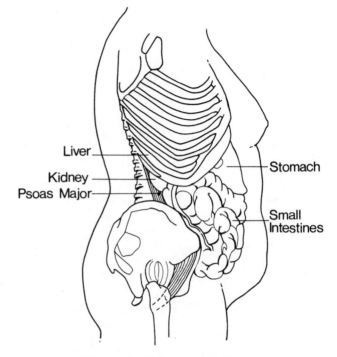

Liver
Kidney
Psoas Major
Stomach
Small Intestines

Figure 3. The psoas shelf.

WHAT DOES THE PSOAS DO?

The most important function of the psoas is to balance and maintain the body parts in the upright position against the force of gravity. As I'll explain in greater detail in Chapter 1, when a segment of the body is out of balance or misaligned and remains that way for a prolonged period of time, the muscles controlling that aspect of posture will contract under the strain and become short and tight. Conversely, the muscle groups working in opposition to the tightened muscles will compensate by stretching. Muscles under prolonged stretch become weak and lose their tone, much as a rubber band stretched past its limit will lose its elasticity. When the psoas muscle group is misaligned or off balance, the muscles in the lower back become short and tight and the abdominal muscles in the front of the torso become stretched and lose their tone. Problems then arise when we try to initiate or sustain movement of those muscles that are already in a state of contraction.

They respond inefficiently, and the result is poor posture, strain on the lower back, and sagging abdominal muscles. A contracted psoas can have far-ranging effects on the body; by throwing the body out of alignment, it can cause problems in the hips, knees, and eventually the upper back, neck, feet, and ankles.

The direct or indirect muscular imbalances that a shortened psoas can affect are many. According to Dr. Michele's theory, it can be the hidden culprit in hip dislocation of a newborn; a toddler's difficulty in learning to walk; "growing pains" in adolescence; back pain in adults; or foot problems throughout life. A malfunctioning psoas muscle can also aggravate such conditions as asthma, circulatory problems, cerebral palsy, emphysema, kidney trouble, menstrual irregularity, and varicose veins. Many of these serious disorders that are aggravated by muscle imbalance can be treated and the painful symptoms alleviated and cured. Obesity and pregnancy can put abnormal pressure on the psoas shelf and increase the pelvic tilt, which produces lower back pain. These problems can often be prevented or corrected by elongating and stretching the shortened, tightened psoas.

The failure to understand the importance of the psoas muscle has led to two popular misconceptions about proper posture and lower back trouble. The first misconception is the notion that bad backs are "weak" and require "strengthening." In fact, to function more effectively most bad backs require lengthening and stretching rather than building and tightening. The already-shortened lower back pulled forward by gravity is relieved of compression when the psoas is properly stretched. The lengthening of the psoas allows for the proper placement of the pelvis to support the spine and provides better posture and alignment for injury prevention.

The second popular misconception concerns proper posture. Many people with poor posture think that their sagging abdomens are simply the result of excess flab. This is only part of the problem. For many people the "potbelly" is a consequence of giving in to the pull of gravity and allowing the tummy to drop forward. This causes the pelvis to tilt forward and the lower back to compress, which in turn shortens the psoas and makes normal postural alignment impossible. This continuous passive tension can produce permanent structural changes in the muscle. When this is the case and a person attempts the wrong type of "stomach strengthening" exercises, he or she may actually increase the compression in the lower back and thus make it more difficult to stand properly and achieve a slimmer waistline. Once again, the solution is to lengthen and stretch the psoas muscle group.

The goal of *Good-bye to Bad Backs* is to provide an easy-to-follow series of exercises to help you engage your psoas muscle properly so that it functions at peak performance. When your psoas is in tip-top shape, it can balance the pressures in the abdominal area; facilitate fuller and better breathing; balance and correct the posture of the spine and pelvis; help you attain a fitter, trimmer appearance; and—best of all—help you say good-bye to the bad back blues.

HOW I DEVELOPED MY PROGRAM FOR LOWER BACK PAIN

I had been an aspiring dancer since I was five years old. When I was twenty-two years old, I was in an automobile accident, which seriously injured my back and affected its flexibility.

Since performing, choreographing, and teaching dance was my chosen career, I had to learn how to accept my limitations and to make modifications in my dance technique. I had to learn how to use my body efficiently and properly so that it could continue to work for me. I took ballet class with the kinesiologist Raoul Gelabert and alignment class with Zena Rommett. I also went to doctors, chiropractors, applied kinesiologists, and massage therapists for some relief from my back pain. But nothing seemed to offer the *consistent* relief that my own stretching exercises did.

I had done some research on back exercises and integrated that with my knowledge of Ideokinesis, the study of dynamic alignment and movement patterns. Then, after studying anatomy with Irene Dowd and attending the Danceclinic sponsored by the Center for Dance Medicine in New York City under the directorship of Dr. Richard Bachrach, I came to understand the importance of a properly functioning psoas.

Now I want to share the secret of the psoas with you. In the following pages I have designed five simple, easy-to-follow thirty-minute workouts that use the principles of Ideokinesis, imagery, stretching and strengthening, and postural alignment to engage the psoas properly and make it flexible, strong, and healthy. This book will benefit in particular five groups of people:

- the average person with lower back pain
- the overweight person
- the pregnant woman
- people with musculoskeletal injuries
- dancers and athletes

If you're an average person with lower back pain, my basic workouts in Chapter 4 will show you how to stretch your lower back and psoas and strengthen your abdominals.

In Chapter 5 I'll discuss more far-reaching exercise programs—such as low-impact aerobics—that will help you keep your body slim and strong. If you're overweight, the extra weight may be pulling your abdomen forward while tilting your spine into a "swayback." The result is poor body alignment that can cause lower back pain and added stress on your joints. In addition to my basic workout and a sound exercise program, you can also use the diet tips in Chapter 5 to help you burn off that extra weight—and say good-bye to the bulging belly blues.

If you're a pregnant woman, you know that the added weight can pull your spine out of alignment, causing lower back pain. In Chapter 6, I'll explain how the pull of gravity affects your pelvis and its contents, and I'll show you exercises tailored especially for pregnant women. These exercises can relieve lower back strain and help pregnant women achieve healthier, happier deliveries.

People who have sustained musculoskeletal injuries must be especially protective of their bodies. In Chapter 7, I'll discuss some of the more common back conditions and how to treat them.

Chapter 8 will help you put the principles of proper body mechanics to use in your daily activities. It will show you how to protect your lower back while doing such ordinary activities as sitting, picking up heavy objects, resting in bed, and so on.

Dancers will be the specific focus of Chapter 9, with visualization exercises and release activities designed to aid in conditioning and injury prevention.

MAKING IT WORK

In my experience, most exercise programs fail because individuals lack motivation. There are several reasons why motivation runs dry:

- the misconception that exercise is too time-consuming and has no place in a busy schedule
- failure to understand the benefits of the exercises
- failure to experience the benefits of exercises because of incomplete or poor instruction.

It is my hope that this book will inspire and motivate all of you who suffer from lower back pain to incorporate exercise into your daily schedules by showing you how to exercise efficiently without injury, by helping you understand the exercise rationale, and by leading you to experience its benefits through thorough and accessible instruction.

IMPORTANT: As with any new fitness regimen, you should consult your physician before beginning my program. It is especially important for you to work with your physician to make sure you don't have a lower back pain problem that requires surgery or that would otherwise make it inadvisable for you to follow the exercises in this book.

Have you stretched your psoas today?

NOTES TO THE INTRODUCTION

1. Morris, A., "Program compliance key to preventing low back injuries," *Occup Health Safety*, March 1984, 44–47.
2. Gyntelberg, F., "One year incidence of low back pain among male residents of Copenhagen, aged 40–59," *Danish Medical Bulletin*, 1974: 21:30–36.
3. *National Center for Health Statistics*, "Limitation of activity due to chronic conditions," United States, 1969 and 1970; 1973: 10(80): 1–54.
4. Orthopaedic Scientific Update: A special report on the scientific sessions of the 51st annual meeting of the American Academy of Orthopaedic Surgeons, *Ortho Nursing*, 1984: 3(2): 47–48.
5. Arthur C. Klein and Dava Sobel, *Backache Relief* (New York: Signet Books, New American Library, 1986).
6. Arthur A. Michele, *Iliopsoas* (Springfield, Illinois: Charles C. Thomas, 1962, p. 4).

Better Posture Means Better Health

Since this is not a textbook, I won't attempt to present an exhaustive discussion of anatomy and kinesiology (the study of mechanics in relation to movement). But in order for you to understand what causes back pain and how to relieve and prevent it, you need to know a little more about the structure and function of the musculoskeletal system. For this reason, allow me to expand on the material I introduced previously.

THE SPINE

The bones of the skeleton form the framework of the body, its joints permit movement, and muscles do the moving.

The backbone of the skeletal system, the spine, is flexible and movable. Structurally strong, it reflects the dynamic movement of the human body. The spine not only supports the body and all its organs, it also moves constantly. Every activity, even breathing, demands movement of the spine and ribs and attachments. The spine gives the human structure both strength and agility.

The spine consists of an S-shaped column of bones called vertebrae. Vertebrae are separated by disks, cushions of connective tissue and cartilage that serve to absorb the shock and impact of body weight as you move. Tough, fibrous ligaments run between the vertebrae and bind them together. Although the ligaments of the spine stabilize it and prevent excessive motion, they do not keep the spine upright. Muscles provide the major support for the spine, keeping it erect and in balance. In particular, the psoas, the abdominals, and the muscles of the back support the spine in the vertical position.

Proper alignment of the spine is important for three reasons: First, the spine encloses a major segment of the central nervous system, the spinal cord. The spinal cord travels from the medulla oblongata at the base of the brain down through the back of the vertebrae in the vertebral canal. Nerves branch out from the spinal cord to different parts of the body. If the vertebrae are pulled out of alignment, they may exert pressure on the nerves in the spinal cord, causing pain or interfering with the ability of a nerve to conduct impulses.

Second, as the vertebrae move, they exert pressure on the disks, the shock absorbers between the vertebrae. Too much pressure from misalignment can cause a disk itself to press against a nerve, which results in sciatica, or lower back pain.

Third, as one part of the spine moves in one direction, another part of the spine must move in an opposing or balancing direction. One misalignment leads to another and one muscle group must compensate for a poorly functioning group, thus affecting the relationship and function of all the organs within the torso.

Mobility of the spine is essential for good posture. The spine has many small joints, and every joint has to be movable in order to stay lubricated. The joints secrete lubrication in the form of synovial fluid even if they are only moved once a day. If the joints are not moved at all, their lubrication runs dry and they feel stiff.

Any twisting or releasing movement can open up a space between the vertebrae and thus cause the synovial fluid to be secreted again, keeping the joints lubricated. (The sound you hear when you "crack" your neck or your knuckles is a vacuum pop that occurs in joints that haven't been moved for a while. The joint acts as an amplification chamber for "gas bubbles.")

Therefore, it is easy to understand that daily movement or exercise is essential in the preventive care for the back.

MUSCLES

The body is built on basic engineering principles. The skeleton is a series of moving parts with bones as the levers and muscles to pull them and make them move. The function of muscles throughout the body has direct and indirect effects on the lower back. If there is something wrong with the attachment of a muscle, or if a muscle is too short or too rigid, stress and strain on the joint result. This leads to improper muscle functioning, which produces bad posture, which in turn causes aches and pains in the back.

Both muscular action and the number of calories metabolized determine whether body weight will remain constant or not. It is muscular action, however, that determines whether healthy circulation will be maintained. Muscular use of the legs pumps blood back to the heart. And the heart itself, which is a muscle, is affected by muscular activity, which trains the heart to beat more efficiently. In our sedentary society, decreased muscular use leads to muscular deterioration. Weakened muscles have less bulk and less oxygen and become flabby and incapable of vigorous or sustained activity. Any unusual exertion puts them under strain, which can result in pain. This increases the likelihood of lower back problems.

Muscles are contractile and exert pull on the tendons and bones to which they are attached. As long as muscles alternately lengthen and contract as the body moves, tendons and ligaments will remain at their normal length and connective tissue will not shrink. But if a joint is maintained in one position for a prolonged period of time, the muscles won't exert any pull on the tendons. This causes the connective tissues on the concave side (inside curve) of the joint to shorten and those on the convex side (outside curve) to lengthen. Overstretching of connective tissues causes the muscles to weaken.

Whenever improper alignment causes excessive pressure

to be exerted on one side of a joint the result is increased wear and tear on the overburdened side, which produces pain. The pain, however, may be reflected in more than that one place because of the muscular attempts at compensation. For example, an individual who continually slumps forward and becomes round-shouldered may experience pain not only in the upper back but in the lower back as a result of the increased compensatory curvature of the lower back. Poor posture, a weak musculature, or any abnormal strain on the joints can have serious ramifications, from nagging lower back pain to osteoarthritis.

Muscles are paired in their action; when one muscle contracts or shortens, its opposite must relax. Muscular imbalance occurs when one muscle group cannot function properly and other muscles compensate for this deficiency.

This is true for the lower back and the abdominal muscles. In order for the abdominal muscles to shorten and contract, their opposite muscle group, the lower back, must be able to lengthen. If, however, the muscles of the lower back are unable to lengthen because of the downward pull of the pelvis, the abdominal muscles will not be able to shorten and contract fully and the back will become compromised.

People with back pain tend to place all the blame on their back muscles, which seems logical since that's where they feel the pain. But they need to recognize that the pain is there because weak, overstretched abdominals and a shortened, tightened psoas have put an excessive workload on the muscles of the back.

Despite the many possible causes of backache, the problem in the great majority of backaches lies with the muscles. Muscles and tissues that become either overstretched and weak or shortened and tightened are unable to perform properly and are vulnerable to injury.

Muscle Spasm

The most frequent immediate cause of acute backache pain is spasm, an involuntary muscular contraction. The spasm is actually a protective mechanism. If there is an injury or a great amount of strain on a joint, the muscles surounding it contract to act as a protective splint and will go into spasm.

You may have noticed this reaction when you try to do too many exercise repetitions or perform an activity that you don't often do. The adjacent muscles may also go into spasm in an attempt to protect the strained muscle and prevent further damage. A spasm can be very painful, and the area becomes tender and swollen.

Under ordinary circumstances, a muscle contracts and rebounds quickly, and the capillaries of the circulatory system can easily transport oxygen and nourishment to the muscle cells and remove its waste products. But when a muscle remains in spasm, the capillaries are closed, and the exchange of materials cannot normally take place. The waste products, which include lactic acid, produce pain when they accumulate in the muscle, resulting in soreness. This is also the familiar "burn" you feel when you overexercise.

Muscle spasm can be caused by an injury, excessive physical strain, or even by emotional tension. Muscle tension is a normal biological response to emotional tension. We have evolved elaborate mechanisms that make it possible for us to respond to emergencies. When we feel threatened, many of our physiological systems are affected. Our respiration increases, our blood pressure rises, our glands begin to secrete hormones, and our muscles prepare us to fight or flee.

Of course, in our civilized society we can seldom fight or flee in most situations. Whether we're having an argument with the office supervisor, watching a scary movie, or in any other tense situation, our bodies may be prepared to take physical action, but for whatever reason, we may not be able to act on it. So we suppress our fear. Perhaps we hunch up our shoulders; as anger is squelched, we may pull and hold our heads back. In short, we build up emotional tension. This tension must somehow be released for the body systems to function optimally.

The release of this tension is important because a muscle must be able to relax easily as well as contract smoothly to maintain full and efficient function. Failing this, jerky and uncoordinated movement can result in injury. Physical exercise provides an excellent outlet for the release of muscular and emotional tension. Exercising helps to dissipate tension in a properly channeled, productive way.

POSTURE AND ALIGNMENT

Now that you understand the basic functions of the muscles and spine, let's integrate them into a broader picture of body posture and alignment and the role of a healthy psoas.

Some people slouch, some people contort their bodies, and some people just drag themselves around. The daily stresses of living are reflected in the way we stand, move, and use our bodies. Incorrect posture can cause a variety of organic as well as musculoskeletal problems.

Posture is the relative arrangement of the different parts of the body. Posture is considered good if the body uses a minimum expenditure of energy to maintain the best balance in its many positions, at rest or in motion. Posture, or standing alignment, is the point of departure for every position and movement that you take during your life. Posture is the reflection of the way you use your body, of how various muscle groups are functioning, and that function is directly related to overall health and fitness. Without balanced alignment it would be impossible to achieve grace, beauty, and efficiency of your body during movement. When alignment is poor, your body moves with strain and difficulty.

Posture is the expression of equilibrium and balance of the body. Posture is an active, dynamic process. It is the result of many involuntary reflexes that interact to keep the body erect and vertical. Continuous and harmonious cooperation of numerous muscles is essential to keep the spine in its normal position. Posture is the result of an interdependency and mutual interaction of nervous impulses and muscular tonicity.

Posture Check

In mechanical terms, normal posture is based on the relationship of the spine to the gravitational line (see Figure 4). Posture depends on a system of balances. It is determined by the alignment of the vertebral column and the lower extremities.

Observe that the spine has four curves. There are forward (concave) curves at the neck and lower back and backward (convex) curves at the center back and sacrum. These curves are normal and give strength, mobility, and resilience to the spine so that it can absorb impact. Any attempts to flatten the

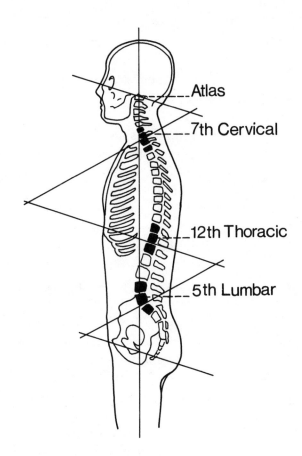

Atlas

7th Cervical

12th Thoracic

5th Lumbar

Figure 4. Postural alignment.

curves place strain and tension on the ligaments and muscles of the lower back. On the other hand, some of the curves of the back, if poorly aligned, may become overly accentuated. When this occurs the spine does not transfer the weight of the body efficiently, making all movement more difficult.

A qualified physician or movement specialist can easily check your posture to see if your body is properly aligned. From observing a person's alignment, a skilled practitioner can predict with reasonable accuracy the stress areas predisposed to injury and degeneration. Here's a method to check yourself:

Have a friend take a picture of you standing in profile. On viewing the photograph, place a dot at the level of your ear, your shoulders, your hip, the front of your knee, and the front of your ankle. Now connect all the dots with a straight line. If one of the dots does not line up and connect with the others, that body part is considered to be out of alignment.

Alternatively, stand sideways in front of a mirror. Check your profile—or have a friend check for you—and try to determine visually which of your body parts fall in front or behind the imaginary line described previously.

The Psoas as Postural Hero

A human is a biped standing erect on two legs. Although the erect position offers the advantages of agility, leverage, and mobility, it also creates certain structural stresses. The body is subject to the force of gravity and the strain of maintaining constant balance.

Posture depends not only on the form of the spine but also on the position of the pelvis. The primary function of the spine is to protect the spinal cord and to maintain the upright position. The pelvis is the base on which the entire spinal column is supported. Because the spine is connected to the pelvis by the sacroiliac joint, the position of the spine is intimately associated with that of the pelvis. Therefore, any change in the position of the pelvis will have an effect on the posture of the spine.

It is impossible to speak of the alignment of the pelvis, lower back, and abdominal areas separately. They are interdependent. When one moves, the others must follow.

When standing in correct alignment, the crest bones of the pelvis should be perpendicular to the ground rather than tilted forward or back. The normal inclination of the pelvis creates a slight concave curve in the lumbar spine (lower back), which in turn balances the convex curve of the thoracic vertebrae (rib cage). These balancing curves are necessary for shock absorption.

The proper placement of the pelvis is determined by the flexibility or rigidity of the psoas, and the psoas is consequently the key to proper body alignment. Recall that the psoas originates in the lower back at the lumbar vertebrae and extends through the abdomen and over the brim of the pelvis to the front of the torso, where it attaches to the inner part of the upper thigh. Its normal function is involved with the entire working of the pelvic area, hips, and back. It is the most important muscle in the pelvic area because it is the closest to the center of gravity and has the best mechanical advantage. To put it simply, the psoas connects the back of you to the front of you. It also stabilizes the spine and pelvis to effect the equilibrium of the spinal curves, and it acts as a shelf to support seven-eighths of the weight of the abdominal contents.

When this primary postural muscle group is shorter and tighter than it should be, it can pull everything out of whack. It can result in extreme lumbar lordosis, or "swayback." In this case, a tight psoas causes the connective tissues in the back of the spine to shorten because of the excessive lumbar lordosis while the abdominal muscles in front become stretched and weakened. The belly sags forward, and so the muscles of the lower back have to work harder to compensate. This increased compression in the lower back causes excessive wear and tear on the joints of the spine because of the inequitable distribution of work. A malfunctioning psoas can also cause "round shoulders." Or, if it's tight and contracted on just one side, the psoas can throw that side of the body out of alignment and cause the other side to strain by overcompensating for this one-sided pull (see Figure 5 on page 20). If the lateral curve created by this pull is more than thirty degrees, it is called scoliosis. The following photographs from Dr. Arthur Michele's book, *Iliopsoas*, show a dramatic change in the spine of a patient with a scoliotic curve after three weeks of derotation exercises and stretches for the psoas.

Posture and Your Health

The most obvious benefits of good posture are biomechanical efficiency and physical comfort. Yet, because of the interrelationship of the structural (bony) and the functional (organ) systems of the body, posture can affect your overall health. As I've mentioned, poor posture compresses the lungs as well as other vital organs of the body, interfering with the body's natural resistance to disease. It can also contribute to shallow breathing, a cramped chest cavity, faulty digestion, poor elimination, lack of energy, and reduced coordination.

Barely perceptible changes in the positioning of the joints and of body segments to each other can dramatically alter optimal mechanical efficiency. Over a period of months or years, the body will be molded in a new image, with a different

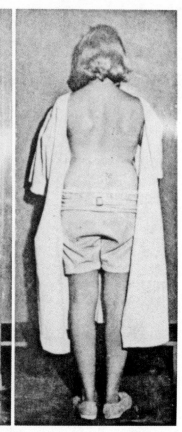

From Arthur A. Michele, *Iliopsoas*, 1962. Courtesy of Charles
C. Thomas, Publisher, Springfield, Illinois.

**Figure 5. A tightened psoas can
cause postural misalignment.**

internal kinesthetic sensibility and relationship to the envi-
ronment.

People with good posture stand taller and look better. Posture affects your image as others see you and as you see
yourself. It reflects your personality, your confidence, your

attitude, and your health. There is also an interrelationship between how you stand, sit, and walk and how you feel.

Understanding why you have poor posture is the first step to correcting it. You may have some congenital problem (one that you were born with) that predisposes you to moving or standing in a certain way. Or you may have the habit of hunching your shoulders in response to a loud, startling noise, or hollowing out your chest when someone yells at you. Or you may have daily working or living habits that cause you to use your body incorrectly. For example, you may always carry your shoulder bag on the same shoulder, or you may always stand with your weight on one leg or you may sit in a chair without proper support.

Many postural problems can be remedied unless there is an anatomical (structural deformity) or pathological (disease-caused) disturbance. Check with your physician to rule out these possibilities. If your poor body alignment and consequent lower back pain are due to a poorly functioning psoas, you can learn to retrain that muscle group to bring it back into shape.

Many people try to correct the muscular imbalance that results from a poorly functioning psoas by using methods that can do more harm than good. For example, constantly holding or squeezing the buttock muscles to achieve pelvic alignment creates chronic tension and makes it difficult to keep your pelvis aligned while you are moving. It also uses up much more energy than is necessary. And trying to flatten your lower back or tuck your pelvis under puts you in an unnatural posture that makes it difficult to work efficiently.

Poor alignment of the lower back and pelvis creates unbalanced tension that can lead to severe back injury. In order to attain good alignment of the pelvis, it is essential that the psoas, the lower back, and the buttocks be capable of relaxing. Only then can realignment work begin. As I'll explain in the next chapter, this is best accomplished by the type of alignment exercises that strive to alter neuromuscular habits through the use of imagery.

2

Relaxation and Stress Reduction

The first step in learning how to care for your lower back is to learn relaxation techniques for stress reduction and increased mobility. The primary technique that you will use for this purpose will be Ideokinesis, aided by proper breathing techniques, which will alter your neuromuscular patterning. What this means is that you will learn to relax by using visualizing and breathing techniques that will begin to change the way you use your body.

Butterflies in the stomach, tension headaches, gastrointestinal problems, high blood pressure, increased heart rate, backache—all are physical signs of twentieth-century stress. The stress reaction fight or flight occurs automatically when we feel threatened. It is a self-protective mechanism that is essential to survival. Over a period of time, this reaction can take its toll. We can learn, however, techniques to reduce stress.

Dr. Herbert Benson, a cardiologist associated with the Harvard Medical School and Beth Israel Hospital in Boston, has been using his "relaxation response" techniques to treat patients with high blood pressure. Stress keeps our muscles in a constant state of tension. However, we can learn to reduce stress by combining some relaxation and visualization techniques with our workouts to get rid of that tension backache.

You can also reduce stress through the physical release of exercise. Exercise can be a very therapeutic means of working off negative feelings. Moderate exercise prompts the release of endorphins from the brain, which have the effect of a natural tranquilizer. The release of endorphins accounts for the "runner's high," the exhilarating, pleasant feeling one gets after a vigorous workout. It is speculated that the endorphin release causes many people to become "addicted" to exercise. They become "dependent" on exercise and feel out of sorts or uncomfortable if they don't exercise. In fact, you may find yourself "hooked" on the exercises for your back in this book. My students have told me that if they miss one day of stretching they can feel the difference in their level of tension and muscular dissatisfaction. They feel that one of the side benefits of the bad-back workout is a great feeling of relaxation and dissipation of tension along with the physical rewards.

RELAXATION

Daily stress produces a high level of arousal that affects everyday bodily functions. Prolonged periods of stress lead to chronic stimulation, then to exhaustion, and eventually to illnesses such as a cold, tension headache, or lower back pain. The debilitation stems from a reduced resistance that is caused by increased levels of stress. We deplete what physiologists call our "adaptive energy." Eventually you "give out" in those areas that are your weakest and most vulnerable.

The daily relaxation habit can assist your body in breaking the circuit of stress naturally by providing the body with a compensatory period known as the "parasympathetic rebound." That means it provides a reversal of the arousal state to enable the body to recharge and rest. Then later, when you encounter the next stressful situation, you're in better control. Your ability to cope will be replenished.

The "relaxation response" is opposite to the typical stress reaction, but it does not occur automatically. It must be developed and practiced. Its benefits include decreased blood pressure and heart and respiration rates, reduced body metabolism and blood flow to the muscles, and increased alpha brain waves, which are associated with feelings of well-being and relaxation. These benefits continue as long as the "relaxation response" is practiced regularly, but they disappear with the cessation of its practice.

Relaxation Response

Find a quiet spot where you will not be disturbed for twenty minutes.

POSITION: Lie supine, with your knees bent and with your legs up on a chair.

ACTIVITY:

1. Close your eyes. Concentrate on your breathing. Allow your lips to part slightly to permit the breath to flow freely. Each time you exhale, allow a sound to occur. Keep your attention focused on your breathing. Listen to the sounds as they fall in and out of your body. Each exhalation sends out tense, jittery feelings. In this relaxed state, a particular thought or feeling may demand attention. Allow it to flow by as if it were on a movie screen. Just try to experience the calm, the relaxation that comes from breathing deeply.

2. Become aware of any "holding" or unnecessary "tightening." Direct your thoughts to a particular tight spot and with each exhalation visualize that spot "melting like butter" until it dissipates.

IMAGERY:

3. Visualize yourself in your favorite relaxation place such as the beach, the mountains, your bed, and so on. Picture yourself there, relaxing and enjoying yourself.

4. Visualize yourself in a positive state. See yourself pain-free, coping easily and without effort. Tell yourself that when you open your eyes, you will continue to have these thoughts and feelings throughout the day.

As you practice this exercise, try the following variations. Imagine:

- My right arm is very heavy.
- My legs are very warm.
- My "center" is warm and glowing.
- My forehead is pleasantly cool.
- My pulse is calm and strong.
- My breathing is calm and regular.

I have just explained the benefits of relaxation in reducing stress. But relaxation is an essential component in stretching muscles. You cannot stretch a muscle if it is not relaxed.

Imagine that the muscle is like a rubber band. If the rubber band is taut, it has no give. On the other hand, if the rubber band is loose, it can stretch easily. The same is true for your muscles. If they are taut as a result of chronic tension and continued misuse, they cannot move, much less stretch. But if the muscle is relaxed and pliable, it can move, which means it can be stretched and strengthened. So for our purposes, if we can learn to relax and let go of unconscious tension, we can stretch our psoas and lower back and build strength in the abdominal muscles in order to prevent lower back pain. The next section on neuromuscular patterning explains how these changes will happen in your body.

NEUROMUSCULAR PATTERNING

From the day we begin moving, we determine our neuromuscular patterns. *Neuromuscular patterning* means that movement occurs as a result of an impulse from the central nervous system, which then transforms electrochemical energy into kinetic or mechanical energy in order to produce the desired movement. A good example of neuromuscular patterning is when we learn how to type. At the start, we "hunt and peck" for the proper key, and after finding it, we strike it. As we practice and become more proficient, we no longer have to look for the keys, because our fingers "remember" where they are. After a while, the entire process becomes automatic and we don't have to think about it at all. This kinesthetic, or movement-learning, experience is called neuromuscular patterning.

Because of the dominance of one of the hemispheres of the brain, as we develop we begin making certain movement choices, such as whether to use the right or left hand as we reach out for something. With each choice and its repetition, our movement vocabulary becomes "fixed." More and more, these choices feel comfortable and "natural" to us even though they may be inefficient. For example, we might find it more "natural" to stand in the swayback position rather than in a properly aligned position. When we discover that our posture is not serving us well and then decide to make positive changes and aspire to the ideal, we may find it difficult and uncomfortable. It will feel "unnatural" because it is not part of our usual or regular movement repertoire.

When a posture is set, the muscles and joints become locked into habitual movement responses, and therefore there are fewer movement choices that the body is capable of making. Yet unconscious habits may involve undue muscular tension and can cause misalignment and prevent free, natural use of the body.

When we consciously begin to try to change our posture, we bring all of our old patterns of movement into play as well. It has been proved that neuromuscular changes can occur much more accurately and directly when they are not active but passive—that is, using imagery rather than new physical actions. With imagery, the thought travels from the brain through the central nervous system affecting a change in the musculature. That is what Ideokinesis is all about.

IDEOKINESIS

What is Ideokinesis? *Ideo* means "idea" or the stimulator of the process; *kinesis* means the physical movement induced by stimulation of the muscles. Ideokinesis is the term Dr. Lulu Sweigard coined to describe the work she did in neuromuscular patterning, which is aimed at improving dynamic alignment and movement patterns. She described Ideokinesis as visualized movement without conscious voluntary action.

The Concept of Ideokinesis

Mabel Ellsworth Todd, who was on the faculty of Teachers College at Columbia University, presented a dynamic theory of the movement process and a new means of dealing with movement training and neuromuscular reeducation that used the power of the mind. She insisted that the visualizations be based on factual images. She invented movement images based on lines of energy as the body performed simple actions or changed positions.

Todd recognized the importance of breathing in facilitating the coordination of movement and created simple games to help the student become aware of his or her breathing patterns. Todd's work was then further developed by two of her students, Barbara Clark and Dr. Lulu Sweigard.

Barbara Clark practiced Ideokinetic technique in her own studio and wrote several books based on her work, one of which is *How to Enjoy Sitting, Standing and Walking*. Andre Bernard, her student and colleague, collaborated with her on some of this work and continues to teach Ideokinesis at New York University.

Sweigard based her work on a scientific study of anatomy, biomechanics, and neurophysiology. Her method of movement reeducation, Ideokinesis, is described fully in *Human Movement Potential: Its Ideokinetic Facilitation*, published in 1974. Ideokinesis is probably the most familiar of the movement-reeducation systems among dancers, because Sweigard taught for many years in the dance department at the Juilliard School.

She described Ideokinesis as visualized movement without conscious voluntary direction or action. Not imposing your old movement habits during this process is the key concept of her method. Sweigard believed, based on her study, that if you concentrate on the image of the movement, the central nervous system can choose the most efficient neuromuscular coordination for its performance. Visualization is a way of "warming up" the neurological pathways. Above all, the student must avoid interfering with this imagined movement by using voluntary muscular action. You *think* it, but don't *do* it.

The images Sweigard chose were based on the realities of kinesiological action, which she translated into "lines of action" for the student to visualize. Sweigard believed that once a more balanced and dynamic skeletal alignment is achieved, much of the individual's movement patterning will also improve. The images she used brought about the relaxation that would allow habitually inefficient muscular habits to be replaced by more efficient neuromuscular patterning in the body. The images must be active. You must learn to see the directional line of energy change and unfold in your mind's eye. Eventually, through repetition and conditioning, the transforming experience is triggered simply by the thought and the image is needed less and less to effect a neuromuscular change.

Much of what we know about proper body mechanics and alignment has been allied with the field of dance, which has been a strong force in education for many years. Scientific methods for working with alignment have become increasingly popular in the dance world. The influences of such innovators as Mabel Todd, Lulu Sweigard, Irmgard Bartenieff, Matthias Alexander, and Moshe Feldenkrais have been seminal in the development of effective techniques for teaching proper alignment.

In the old days, the dance teacher would try to correct postural alignment by training the student to hold a new position that looked correct. This approach assumed that the dancer would be able to "feel" the correct new posture after doing it by rote for a period of time.

We now know that this method makes the muscles do too much work. The resulting buildup of constant, unnecessary muscle contractions, called chronic tension, robs the body of needed energy. In a standing posture, the primary function of the muscles is to hold you in balance. The better aligned you are, the less work your muscles have to do. And just as poor alignment causes a buildup of chronic tension, working with too much tension can create alignment problems.

What Todd, Sweigard, Bartenieff, Alexander, and Feldenkrais have contributed to our pool of knowledge is that in order to change old, ingrained movement habits in a permanent way, the brain must develop new neuromuscular patterns and coordination. They discovered that this is best accomplished through the use of imagery and "imagined movement."

Ideokinesis uses imagery directed by lines of directional energy, which assists you in restructuring your own body from within by using proper breathing techniques, tactile or verbal cues, deep and slow movements, and barely perceptible shifts in structural balance.

Despite the fact that the body seeks balance and harmony, subtle muscular imbalances do occur between the levels of the body. In general, we're preoccupied with the outer level of muscles in our body—the biceps, pectorals, abdominals, gluteals. We target our exercise at them in the hope of improving our physical appearance, and the result is that these muscles are overworked, overused, and in a state of chronic tension. Meanwhile, at a deeper level, muscles such as the psoas and those supporting the spine and rib cage can become atrophied from lack of use.

It is the purpose of this book to engage and restore the psoas muscle group to its best mechanical advantage and reactivate its proper function by the use of imagery and gentle stretching exercises.

MAKING CHANGES HAPPEN

1. Remember: Your goal is to alter the way muscles pattern themselves to produce movement.
2. Since muscle action is neurologically controlled, changes involve alterations in the functioning of brain networks. The way you *think* about a movement or exercise can assist you in performing or executing it well.
3. Become aware of your own "self-use," your own patterns of movement, so that change can take place.
4. Use this awareness to develop your own techniques based on the sound principles of this program.
5. Learn that "effort" sometimes means doing nothing! You can facilitate positive changes with "effortless effort."
6. Accept the fact that this is a process that will take time. Be patient. If you have been standing in a particular posture for twenty years, don't expect the changes to occur in one or two sessions. But, remember, with each repetition, the new movement choices will become easier and more "natural" to you.

THE USE OF IMAGERY

As a result of movement research, more movement practitioners are aware of the importance of accurate visual images in stimulating the desired kinesthetic or movement response. Some of the most poetic images, such as a flowing waterfall or a billowing parachute, have been discovered to be right on target with some of the most recent scientific thinking about how the neurological system functions in motor learning.

Imagery helps a person to relax and concentrate. If you can visualize a body part, you can usually feel it better. In your imagery rehearsal, you mentally experience a movement or activity as though you were actually doing it. The closer you can come to simulating an actual situation, the greater are your chances of developing the skill to perform well in that situation.

PRACTICING VISUALIZING TECHNIQUES

The following techniques will *not* increase muscular strength or cardiovascular fitness. The muscular recoordination that will occur as a result of using these visualizing techniques while concentrating on imagined action will be ease of movement, increased flexibility, and better postural alignment. These techniques have been developed to meet the needs of the majority of people, regardless of special situations and daily activities. Techniques I and II are visualization only. Techniques III, IV and V are visualization and movement.

Points to Remember

1. Full concentration must be given to the exercise itself. The pattern of movement must be learned first.
2. The mind should focus and concentrate on the imagery.
3. Imagined movement should be used both before and during the voluntary movement.
4. Range of motion should be small, and movement must be *slow* in order to allow time for imagined action.
5. The sequence for each exercise should be:
   A. Execution of voluntary movement or exercise.

B. Rest.

C. Imagine the action.

D. Perform the movement while concentrating on the imagery.

E. Rest.

F. Make a mental note of any changes that you experience or feel.

VISUALIZING TECHNIQUES

As in all the movement-reeducation systems, you begin by lying down on the floor—a position that minimizes the effects of gravity on your posture. You may want to use a mat or towel to cushion your body. When your body is in a more relaxed state, you will be able to "give up" and "let go" of old movement patterns. Close your eyes and relax.

I.	*Rest Position with Centered Breathing: The Parachute*
PURPOSE:	To promote relaxation and better alignment and to reduce stress and muscular tension.
POSITION:	Lie supine, with your knees bent and your feet flat on the floor. Rest your arms alongside your body on the floor.
ACTION:	Notice any points of tension in the body or places where your muscles are "holding." Take an ordinary breath and with an easy exhalation feel those tension points release and let go. Repeat this several times.
IMAGERY:	With each inhalation, visualize the rib cage expanding just like a parachute billowing with air. With each exhalation, see the parachute collapse into the center of your body (see Figure 6 on page 32).

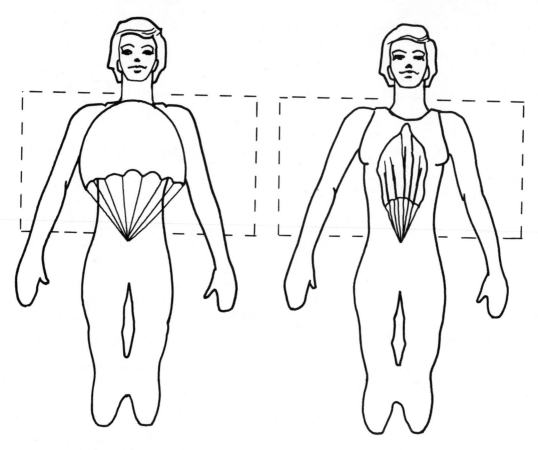

Figure 6. The parachute.

II.　　　　*Lower Back and Spine Release*

PURPOSE:　To release the deep muscles along the spine
and to engage them in subtle movements
with each breath.

POSITION:　Lie supine, with your knees bent and feet
flat on the floor. Rest your arms alongside
your body on the floor.

ACTION:　Take deep breaths that feel three dimen-
sional; feel the torso expand and widen as
though it were a full, round cylinder.

IMAGERY:　See the weight of the pelvis sinking down

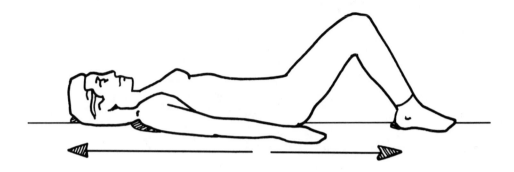

Figure 7. Lower back and spine release.

to your legs as though it were as heavy as an anchor. See all of your vertebrae move away from the pelvis in the opposite direction toward your head. See your head continue floating away from your pelvis (see Figure 7).

III.   *Thigh Flexion*

PURPOSE: To use the abdominal and psoas muscles in their resting length and to improve the efficiency of their coordination.

POSITION: Lie supine, with your knees bent, and feet flat on the floor. Rest your arms alongside your body on the floor.

ACTION: Raise your right thigh toward your chest, letting the foot hang so that it leaves the floor last. The abdominal muscles should be soft and should not bulge up. Repeat with your left thigh.

IMAGERY: See and feel your thighbone as very *heavy*. As you raise it toward your chest, you sense

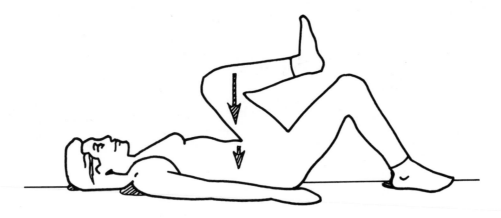

Figure 8. Thigh flexion.

its weight "pouring" down into the hip joint in the pelvis (see Figure 8).

IMAGES FOR PELVIC ALIGNMENT

IV.	*Pelvic Swing*
PURPOSE:	To enable the pelvis to move freely.
POSITION:	Stand with your feet straight ahead and your knees slightly bent.
ACTION:	Place one hand on your abdomen and the other hand on your lower spine. Keep your abdominal and buttocks muscles relaxed. Gently swing your pelvis forward and backward.
IMAGERY:	Imagine that you have a flashlight placed at the level of each hipbone. As you swing your pelvis forward and backward, see the light move from the straight-forward position to upward and then down to the floor (see Figure 9).

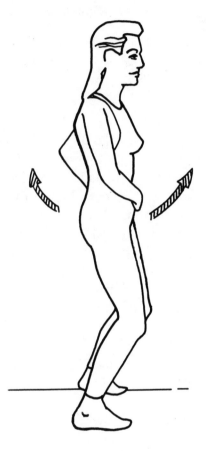

Figure 9. Pelvic swing.

V. *Dinosaur's Tail*

PURPOSE: To engage the abdominal muscles efficiently without tension.

POSITION: Stand with your feet straight ahead and your knees slightly bent.

ACTION: Bend your knees without taking your feet off the floor. Slowly straighten your legs upward. Try not to hyperextend your knees (pushing the knees too far back) because that will cause the pelvis to tip forward. Repeat several times.

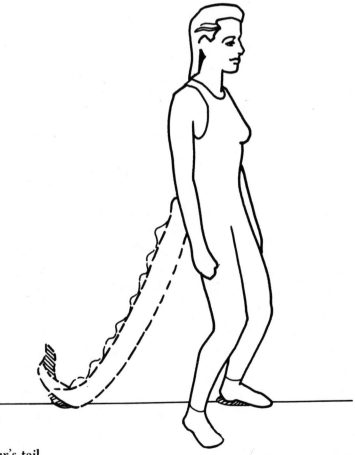

Figure 10. Dinosaur's tail.

Imagine that you have a long dinosaur's tail extended from the end of your tailbone toward the floor. As you straighten upward, continue the image of the weight of the tail dropping down to the floor (see Figure 10).

BREATHING

Breathing is a total body experience. When the diaphragm is allowed to expand fully, its lengthening movement is communicated through the whole spine, from the tailbone to the skull and through the pelvis, legs, and feet. Although the psoas is not a respiratory muscle, its immobility can impede the breathing process. Deep breathing can heal pain, reduce tension, and channel necessary energy into the body.

On inhalation the diaphragm lengthens the thoracic area and increases the circumference of the rib cage. The exhalation phase starts with the pull of gravity on the ribs, which is continued by increased muscular contraction as the exhalation is prolonged.

Breathing is always influenced by postural alignment and the position of the body. The better the alignment, the greater the efficiency.

The person with lower back lordosis (swayback) uses the front half of the diaphragm more than the back half. When he or she breathes, the upper abdomen moves forward, raising the chest upward rather than allowing the rib cage to expand three-dimensionally. The corrective breathing exercise for the shortened lower back is the "centered" breathing exercise, because it conforms with the structure and proper function of the diaphragm.

When breathing is centered properly in the trunk, the abdominal area will noticeably raise up toward the ceiling as the diaphragm places pressure on the abdominal organs. With the exhalation, the abdominal area will sink down toward the floor as the diaphragm pulls up and releases its pressure on the abdominal organs.

Basic Breathing Exercise with Pelvic Tilt

Breathing is an unconscious, automatic act. You don't have to do anything to make it happen, but you can become more aware of it. I'd like you to try an awareness exercise right now to get in touch with and understand this process better.

POSITION: Lie supine, with your knees bent and feet flat on the floor.

ACTION: Close your eyes and place your hands on top of your tummy. Allow yourself to become aware of the breathing process. See how it happens without your doing anything at all. It happens as naturally and unconsciously as digesting your food.

Become aware that your tummy goes up toward the ceiling as you inhale and drops down toward the floor as you exhale.

Step 1:   Exaggerate the normal breathing pattern and really expand your tummy as

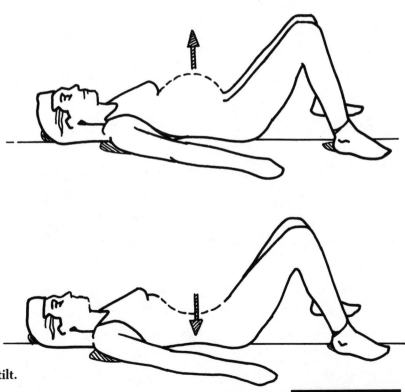

Figure 11.
Basic breathing with pelvic tilt.

you inhale and really press your tummy down to the floor as you exhale. Repeat this several times. Return to normal breathing (see Figure 11).

Step 2: Imagine that you have the face of a clock superimposed on the pelvic area. Six o'clock will be at your tailbone and twelve o'clock will be at the upper rim of the pelvis just behind the belly button. Now do a small rocking motion from 6:00 to 12:00. Rock down to your tailbone, arching your back slightly, and then slowly rock up to 12:00, pressing the lower back flat on the floor. Repeat several times (see Figure 12).

Step 3: Put the breathing and the movement together. Start first with your normal breathing awareness. Then slowly begin to exaggerate your normal breathing until you are really expanding the abdominal area as you inhale and really press your tummy down to the floor as you exhale.

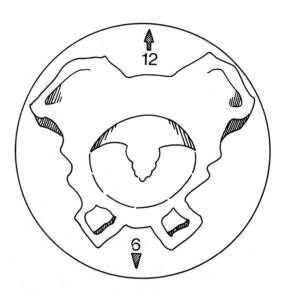

Figure 12. The pelvic clock.

Step 4: Next, add the pelvic tilt. As your tummy expands as you inhale, rock down to your tailbone. As you exhale, press 12:00 (belly button) down to the floor. Repeat several times until you feel that you have integrated the breath and the pelvic tilt as best as you can.

Don't get upset with yourself if you don't master this technique immediately. It generally takes my students several attempts before this becomes comfortable and automatic for them. But stay with it, because it is the basic breathing that we will use in the exercises that follow.

"THINK EXHALE! THE INHALE WILL NATURALLY FOLLOW"

I like to have my students focus on the active out-breath, or exhalation, using abdominal and thoracic muscles to squeeze air from the lungs and create a partial vacuum so that inhalation can take care of itself passively. What you want to do is push the old, stale air out and allow the new fresh air to flow in easily. As you actively force air from the lungs in this way, you flatten the abdominal area down to the floor and tilt the pubic bone up as you tilt the tailbone under.

Your awareness of this integration of movement and breathing with its accompanying source of power and strength while performing your exercises will provide increased stamina and will enable you to perform the exercises in an easier, more relaxed manner.

Physiologists recognize that exhalation facilitates a relaxation response that lowers the blood pressure. Hence, when lifting a heavy weight, you exhale on the exertion to balance the workload. Physiologists also recognize that the heart pumps a greater volume of blood during exhalation than it does during inhalation, increasing the body's oxygen-using potential.

Extensive testing of the technique of emphasizing the exhalation during performance was conducted at the University of Toledo in 1986, where a group of cyclists and triathletes were tested before and after using this breathing technique for one week. Researchers found improved physiological function as related to performance for those test subjects who used the breathing technique. In addition, the test subjects reduced both their blood pressure and pulse rates by 10 to 15 percent while performing at the same work rate. Their oxygen consumption increased, and they were able to burn fats at a slower rate, thus delaying the time of total fatigue.

Exhalation

1. Inhale through your nose and exhale through your mouth, leaving your lips slightly parted.
2. Allow a soft *sss* sound to pass your teeth and your lips as you exhale.
3. *The exhalation is most important.* Don't think about the inhalation. It will happen automatically. (When a child has a temper tantrum and faints because he holds his breath, he will automatically inhale when his body thwarts his conscious, willful action.)
4. It is important to let out as much air as possible during the exhalation because the amount of air left in the lungs from a previous inhalation limits the amount of fresh air that can be taken in during the next inhalation. The body can function for a longer period of time at a level of high activity if as much old air as possible is expelled from the lungs after taking in as much fresh air as possible.
5. The exhalation is important because the more air you expel, the more oxygen you will automatically take in. Also, as you exhale, a physiological relaxation response occurs that lowers your blood pressure. The relaxation response will help you stretch and release a muscle with greater ease, since lactic acid, a metabolic waste product, is then released from the muscle.

Exhalation Imagery 1: **The Human Thermometer**

POSITION: Lie supine, with your knees bent and your feet flat on the floor.

ACTION: Breathe.

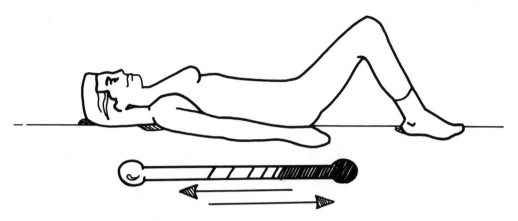

Figure 13. The human thermometer.

IMAGERY: Imagine the breath going up and down the central axis of your body, the front of your spine. See your breath begin at your pelvis and continue up the front of your spine and out through the top of your head. Picture a mercury thermometer. As you inhale, watch the thermometer's mercury go up. As you exhale, watch the thermometer's mercury go down (see Figure 13).

Exhalation Imagery 2: **The Pine Tree**

POSITION: Stand with your hips, knees, and ankles in alignment.

ACTION: Breathe through your central axis. Feel your weight balanced around this central pole. As the axis remains stable, don't allow yourself to give in to gravity; but instead, sense and feel your muscular body draping easily around the central axis. Since your bones will be more closely aligned around its center, your muscles will be able to relax and not work as hard to keep you upright against the pull of gravity.

IMAGERY: Feel that your central axis is like that of a pine tree. Its trunk is firmly based on the ground with energy going up its center, growing taller and taller as the energy flows upward. The branches of the tree slope downward and move freely without effort. Allow your shoulders, arms, and rib cage to hang around your center in a relaxed way (see Figure 14).

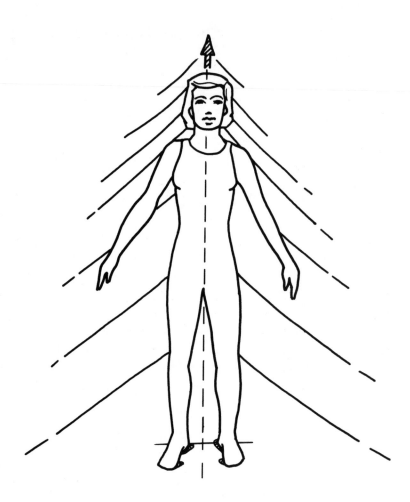

Figure 14. The pine tree.

3

Getting Ready for Your Workout

After you've mastered relaxation technique, the next stage in the rehabilitative process of healing the lower back begins with stretching exercises, followed by muscular strengthening, and, finally, developing habits of proper body mechanics. The most important of the strengtheners is the abdominal series, which will help to support the front of the body and thus enable the back to "let go" and lengthen. Proper body mechanics reduce the physical strain that poor postural habits usually put on the muscles of the back.

STRETCHING

Stretching properly can prevent injury, but it can actually cause injury when done incorrectly. You increase your range of motion when stretching because you actually lengthen and elongate the muscle fibers. When you stretch consistently, you can change the length of the muscle fibers so that they can maintain this increased length.

It is important to note that any pain or discomfort while stretching should be felt in the "belly" of the muscle and not in the tendon or the joint.

Muscles can stretch and return to their original length without damage because they are elastic. Tendons and ligaments, however, are inelastic. Tendons, which attach muscles to bones, can become strained and partially torn when they are over-stretched. This pain or irritation in the tendon is called ten-dinitis. Ligaments stabilize the joints and attach bone to bone. When you stretch a ligament, it can become permanently lengthened and the joint that it is supposed to support be-comes loose and weak. Tendon and ligament injuries take longer to heal than muscle injuries because of their limited blood supply.

The stretch reflex is the body's protective mechanism against trauma and injury. If a muscle is stretched too far, too soon, a message is sent from the brain to pull the muscle back and contract it in order to prevent injury. If you continue to stretch the muscle when this happens, you will be trying to lengthen a muscle that is in the process of shortening. In effect, you and the muscles "have an argument," because double mes-sages are being sent, which results in a cramp that stops all activity. Bouncing while stretching or forcing a muscle to stretch will always trigger the stretch reflex.

Stretching and the Psoas

The primary function of the psoas is to keep you balanced in the upright, vertical position. The action of the psoas brings your thighbone to your torso, or your torso to your thighbone. Therefore, every time you take a step forward to walk or run (bringing your thigh to your torso) or every time you sit down, bend, or sleep (bringing your torso to your thigh), you are using your psoas muscle. It is obvious that we use the psoas muscle constantly.

Whenever you stand upright with poor postural habits (swayback and sagging belly) you are perpetuating the short-ened, tightened psoas. Since the origin of the psoas is in the lumbar spine and its insertion is inside the inner thighbone, it becomes easier to understand that unless these two points are stretched away from each other, the shortening process will continue (see Figure 15). That means that when the psoas is not working, its ability to release, rest, and stretch will be impaired. Remember, an optimally functional muscle must be able to release, to stretch, and to contract for greatest efficiency and power.

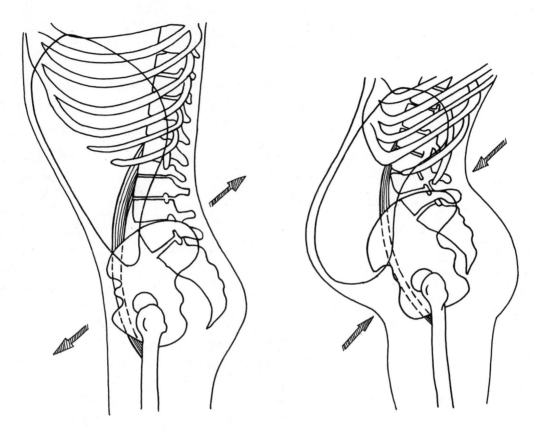

Figure 15. A shortened, tightened psoas creates
a swayback and sagging belly.

**Why You Need to Stretch
the Psoas Muscle:**

- to align the pelvis properly to support the spine.
- to achieve greater stretch and mobility of the muscles of
  the lower back.
- to achieve greater and more "complete strength" of all the
  abdominal muscles (meaning that all of the muscle fibers of
  a particular muscle group will have the potential to be more
  consistently strengthened if the muscle can move through
  a full range of motion).

Even if you exercise regularly, you may not be stretching
your psoas. Walking and running cause great stress to the
psoas. These are weight-bearing activities that bring the leg
to the torso repeatedly. It is the constant repetition, without
variation, that can really cause psoas tightness. Since many

more people are walking and running for their aerobic fitness, I would like to take some time to talk about that.

A healthy body is characterized by balance. Each individual muscle should be equally flexible and strong, as should its opposing muscle. Any time one muscle gets stronger than its counterpart, injury is more likely to occur.

Walking and running are unbalanced activities. Each stride forward is the product of a series of contractions of the Achilles tendon, the calf muscles, the quadriceps, and the psoas.

The psoas muscle shortens every time a runner lifts his or her knee forward in a running stride. This repeated shortening without the opposing action, stretching, will cause the psoas to become shorter and tighter. This means that the psoas will not only be shorter in its resting state, but it will prevent movement around the hip joint. The range of motion will be restricted, and the entire body will be out of balance.

Any tight muscle in the body pulls the connecting bones out of proper alignment; a tight psoas, however, is particularly detrimental because it changes the tilt of the pelvis. As stated previously, the hip is flexed forward by two main muscles, the psoas and the rectus femoris (part of the quadricep group). If these muscles remain shortened, they will pull the pelvis forward. When the pelvis tilts forward, the lower back is contracted, creating an exaggerated curve in the lower spine. The overall effect of this misalignment is one of compensation and compression resulting in lower back pain.

Regular, proper stretching of the psoas can prevent muscle tightness, joint limitation, and misalignment. Therefore, if you are a regular walker or runner, you should stretch the Achilles, the calf, and the quadriceps, but most importantly, the psoas, since it is the major hip flexor that brings the leg to the torso. It's important to stretch after every run or walk. Stretching after exercise gets the kinks out more easily because the body is warmed up and pliable.

When trying to determine the level of stress on the psoas, consider the movements involved in the activity and how often the limbs are used in a particular way. For example, swimming would not be as stressful to the psoas as ballet would be. Swimming is nonweight bearing, and there are a variety of swim strokes that can be used to propel you through the water.

Ballet dancing would be of greater stress to the psoas because it is weight bearing and it uses many of the same gestures to bring the leg to the torso (e.g., Grand Battement) or the torso to the leg (e.g., Porte de Bras). There is greater use against gravity, and therefore, a greater need for stretch. Keep this in mind whenever you exercise—variety of motion and proper stretching will help you get the most out of the activity you choose.

Stretch Your Psoas Daily

Since the psoas is in constant daily use, it is essential to stretch it daily. The time is up to you. If you have a few minutes before you start the day, do it then. Or if you prefer stretches at night, that's fine, too. Just make sure to set a few minutes aside each day to give your psoas a much-deserved release. See page 165 for a quick psoas mini-workout. You may not always have time for a complete workout, but you can always set aside a few minutes for this simple stretching routine.

Points to Remember for Good Stretching

Don't stretch unless you are totally warmed up. When your muscles are cold, they resist stretching. Stretching is really the opposite of warming up. Stretching releases and lengthens the muscles; the warm-up increases heart rate, blood flow, and breathing rates.

Gently ease your body into the stretch position. Remain in this position and relax and breathe. Hold the stretch position for thirty to sixty seconds. Don't push yourself any farther. Just stay there and breathe until your body adjusts. If you feel a *mild* discomfort, this is a "good hurting." Just stay there and relax and breathe. If the pain feels acute and very uncomfortable, this is "bad hurting." Slowly release yourself out of the stretch and stop for the time being.

To increase your range of motion, you must stretch consistently. Once your maximum stretch has been achieved, it takes considerably less effort to maintain.

It is necessary to accept the limits of your own maximum stretch, which is determined by your anatomical structure and the length and position of your ligaments. For example, women usually have an easier time than men stretching in the V-sitting position because their pelvises are wider.

When starting your exercise program, do your exercises slowly. Don't push or force the exercises or bounce while stretching. Use your judgment. If a particular stretch doesn't feel right to you, don't do it. If it feels as though it will take time to work it through, stay with it, relaxing and breathing into the stretch. You will begin to feel your muscle release and let go. You will feel yourself getting close to your goal. Be patient. It will take time.

SUGGESTED MUSIC FOR STRETCHING

I've always found that music is the perfect accompaniment to stretching; it helps soothe and release you and lets you ease into a natural rhythm.

The following composers or musical groups have provided the most suitable music selections for my stretch classes. I offer them only as suggestions; you should feel free to select music that you respond to the most.

- Philip Glass
- Steven Halprin
- Paul Horn
- David Hykes and the Harmonic Choir
- Steve Reich
- Shadowfax
- Andreas Vollenweider
- Windham Hill
- Paul Winter

When choosing music for stretching, you should make sure that the music soothes and relaxes you and that it is slow so that you don't rush through your stretches.

STRENGTHENING

The strength of a muscle is determined by the distance over which it can contract. The longer or more stretched the muscle fibers are, the greater the distance they can contract and the more power they have. This kind of strength is called efficient strength. When the muscles are not stretched, they can only get strong by becoming big and bulky. Efficient strength creates a long slim line in the muscles, which is why a dancer with thin thigh muscles can be much stronger than an athlete who has bulky thighs.

Therefore, you need a balance between stretch and strength. Strengthening your body is important, but without simultaneously stretching your muscles, you will have thick, inefficient muscle with limited range of motion. And conversely, stretching without strengthening to support your flexibility will leave you prone to injury.

WHY AND HOW TO STRENGTHEN THE ABDOMINALS

Skeletal muscle is voluntary contractile tissue that moves your skeleton. There are two functionally different groups of muscles in the body. The outer musculature includes the gluteals, the latissimus dorsi, the trapezius, the pectorals, the rectus abdominus, the biceps, the triceps, the quadriceps, the hamstrings, and the calf. The deeper, inner musculature includes the psoas, the external rotators, the transversus abdominus, the intercostals, and the erector spinae. The larger, overlying musculature is used for flight or fight and moves at a faster rate than the inner musculature. The overdevelopment of these muscles prevents us from experiencing or using the deeper musculature to its fullest degree.

Western culture seems to fixate on the development of the superficial musculature. When we overbuild and tighten our outer musculature ("pecs" and "lats," for example), they become bulky and restricted in range of motion. We build an armor that prevents us from moving fully or using our deeper muscles. And since they are deeper, we don't experience or feel them as we can the outer muscles. We definitely can feel when we are stretching our calf or our hamstring, but we don't feel the psoas stretch in the same way. We experience the stretching of the psoas as the less concrete sensation of "opening up the hip joint" or as a feeling that we are standing

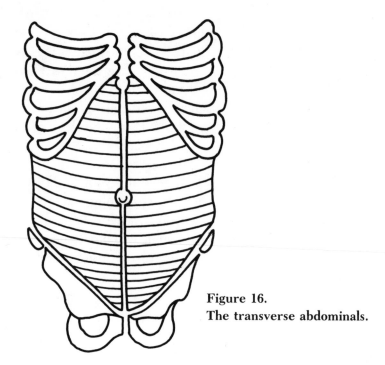

Figure 16.
The transverse abdominals.

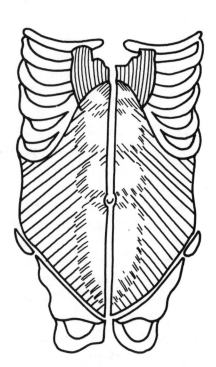

Figure 17. The internal obliques.

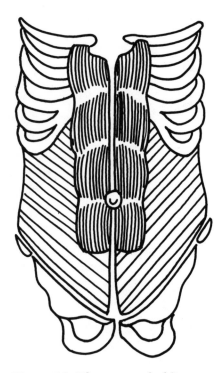

Figure 18. The external obliques
and rectus abdominus.

up straighter and taller. The deeper musculature of the abdominals is the transversus abdominus. Many of the body's vital organs are in the abdominal region. The transverse abdominals protect these vital organs and help to maintain their proper position in the abdominal cavity. They also assist in breathing and elimination.

Using All of the Layers of the Abdominals Really Trims the Tummy

There are four groups of abdominal muscles. They are the transversus abdominus, the internal obliques, the external obliques, and the rectus abdominus. The transverse abdominals start in the back at the spine and wrap around to the front, acting like a "cinch belt" to hold the abdominal contents intact (see Figure 16). The next layer on top of the transversalis are the internal obliques. They, too, start from the spine and wrap diagonally upward to the front and attach to the sternum (see Figure 17). On top of the internal obliques are the external obliques, which start at the spine and move diagonally forward and down to the pubic bone (see Figure 18). They are hip flexors that bring the torso to the legs. The most superficial layer of abdominals is the rectus abdominus. This muscle extends in front from the sternum to the pubis. It brings the torso to the legs.

Perhaps the most important reason that the abdominal region is the first to show deterioration and fat accumulation is that the abdominal muscles are the least-used muscles of the body. Through poor postural habits, our abdominals are constantly being overstretched, and, therefore, they lack muscle tone. When starting an exercise program, people often work only the rectus abdominus (the outer layer of abdominals), rarely engaging the oblique abdominals and never using the transverse abdominals. My exercise program will strengthen all of the deep layers of abdominals.

Many people come to my exercise classes saying that they want to get rid of their flabby tummy. They want a "flatter stomach." First of all, I tell them that their stomach digests their food, and what they're really referring to is their abdominal wall. If they have an overabundance of subcutaneous fat (fat just underneath the skin as opposed to intramuscular fat), they must burn that fat by exercising aerobically and eating properly (see Chapter 6). Second, they must elongate the psoas so that the pelvis can be aligned properly. Finally, they should be doing their abdominal exercises daily at home and not just when they come to class.

When the tone of the abdominal muscles decreases through inactivity, the bulging belly syndrome appears. As muscle tone is lost, the accumulated fat causes the waistline to stretch even further. Poor posture accentuates a pot belly even more. Lack of tone of the abdominal muscles combined with poor posture can add two to three inches to your waist measurement even if you haven't gained a pound.

A vicious cycle occurs when you want to "flatten your tummy" and the psoas is in its shortened state. In this condition, the pelvis is tilted forward, shortening the muscles of the lower back. If the psoas is not stretched, the lower back cannot fully release and lengthen, nor can the abdominals fully shorten and tighten. If the exerciser then proceeds to perform abdominal exercises using only the outer musculature (rectus abdominus), he or she will end up developing a bulging belly, not a flatter tummy.

**How to Perform
Abdominal Exercises**

One of the most important aspects of abdominal exercise is proper breathing. To contract and use the abdominals fully, you must always exhale on the exertion. For example, when you are executing the "crunch" or the "curl-up," you should exhale as you move your torso forward. Inhale as you move your torso back toward the floor. The diaphragm contracts as you exhale and assists the abdominals in their contraction. If you try to inhale as you are contracting your abdominals, you will stretch your diaphragm, preventing full use of all the deep layers of the abdominals.

**How to Begin
the Abdominal Exercises**

1. Stretch your psoas.
2. Focus your attention on deep abdominal breathing.
3. Learn to coordinate the execution of the abdominal exercise with your breathing.
4. Use the image of "hollowing out" the abdominal area or "pressing the belly button down to the floor" on the execution and exhalation.

HOW TO DO YOUR WORKOUT

The exercises for the psoas, lower back, and abdominals are interspersed and are designed to flow in a logical progression from one to the other. Therefore, it is best and easiest to follow the suggested sequence.

Start with Workout #1 and stay with it until you feel that you are sufficiently released in the psoas and lower back. When you need more challenging abdominal exercises, move on to Workout #2. Keep track of your progress and how long it takes you to progress from a particular workout to a more difficult one. Keep track of all your exercise "firsts."

Work-a-Day/Rest-a-Day

Your progress will be determined by the frequency of your workouts. Stretching can and should be performed every day, as can the mild abdominal exercises.

Once you are performing the more difficult abdominal exercises, you should alternate a "heavy day" with a "light day." By that I mean, if you're using five-pound weights as you do the abdominal strengtheners on a Monday and you want to exercise on Tuesday, use no weights on Tuesday.

This is the "work-a-day/rest-a-day" dictum of exercise. You must give the muscles time to recover in order to be stressed to the maximum at the next workout. That recovery time is usually twenty-four to forty-eight hours. In the example above, your next heavy-weight workout should be on Wednesday. However, if you miss your workout on Wednesday, you will begin to regress and lose some of the benefits gained on your workout on Monday. That's why you should try to do your workout at least three to four times per week.

For example, your Workout schedule might look like this:

Monday	Tuesday	Wednesday	Thursday	Friday	Saturday	Sunday
Rest	Stretch/ Workout	Rest	Stretch/ Workout	Rest	Stretch/ Heavy Workout	Stretch/ Light Workout

**Good Hurting
vs. Bad Hurting**

As you begin doing more repetitions and challenging yourself with more difficult abdominal exercises, you may begin to feel a burning sensation in the abdominal area. This is "good hurting." The burn happens when your muscles are beginning to fatigue. However, if you feel a pain of any kind in your back, *stop* what you are doing and either don't do that particular set of abdominal exercises or make some modifications, such as going back to an easier set of abdominal exercises. For example, if you were doing the exercises with your hands crossed on your chest, you might try bringing your hands forward to give you the help of their additional weight going forward. Or you might check your form. Make sure that your belly button is always pressing down to the floor. If you are doing abdominal exercises that require your legs to be extended off the floor in front of you and your lower back comes off the floor to do so, raise your legs higher to the ceiling so that you will be able to keep your lower back flat on the floor.

Pain is your body's way of telling you that something you're doing is not right. Pay attention to that signal and make some modifications. Listen to your body. It will let you know when you are working too hard or when you are not working hard enough. It will let you know when your alignment is off and when you are not getting the proper support to execute the exercise. You are the best friend your body ever had. Take good care of it.

BUILDING RIGHT ATTITUDES ABOUT EXERCISE

A person in pain will do almost anything to alleviate it. As the lower-back-pain sufferer begins to do an exercise program on a regular basis, he or she will find that the pain diminishes or disappears completely. Gradually the person might begin to become negligent about exercising and slip back to old habits and patterns that result once again in the painful lower back syndrome.

The lower-back-pain sufferer must realize that exercise must become a daily habit, an integral part of his or her life-style. My students have told me that sometimes they have to drag themselves to my class because they are so tired. Yet, they all exclaim, "But I knew how good I would feel afterwards." Remind yourself how good you will feel after stretching and exercising. Remember how terrible you feel when you don't stretch and exercise. Your twenty-minute program will be a pleasurable time. It will become a part of your day that you will look forward to. Exercise and stretch because you like to. Then do it for what it does for you, and you'll always have the motivation to do it again and again.

Building Motivation

Every day review the benefits that you will accrue as a result of integrating exercise into your life.

1. Your lower back pain will be lessened or eradicated.
2. You will be able to control your weight without going on a fad diet.
3. You will have more stamina, energy, and greater productivity.
4. You will sleep better and have greater resistance to stress.
5. You will have a more youthful body with good alignment and muscular strength and definition.
6. You will enhance your self-image.

Points to Remember

1. Wear comfortable, nonbinding clothes. During chilly winter days wear warm sweat clothes to keep your muscles from getting too cold. During hot weather wear soft cotton to absorb perspiration.
2. Start slowly. A gentle progress will avoid muscle strain and give your body time to develop the necessary strength to make the exercises more pleasurable and easy to do.
3. Set aside a special time in your day for your exercise program—a time that is yours alone. It can be early morning, before the day begins, or it can be at the end of the day when you can relax. The important thing is to establish a *regular* time, day after day, to exercise.
4. Make a special place for your exercising. Make sure you have enough space to move your arms and legs around

freely. If you don't have carpeting or a thick rug, use an exercise mat to cushion yourself.

5. Set attainable goals. Know your limitations and gear your progress to what your body feels, not to what you *think* you *should* be doing.

6. As muscle strength begins to improve, substitute other exercises with greater strengthening results. Substitution rather than addition won't add time to your workout and will lead to improvement at a faster rate.

7. Focus on your progress. Take before and after photos. Keep notes in an exercise journal to indicate when a particular exercise becomes "easy," and note any exercise "firsts." Use the "Weekly Workout Diary" to help you keep track of your progress. You'll be surprised and delighted at the extent and rate of your improvement.

Exercise Do's and Don'ts

1. DO start your exercise workout with a warm-up.

2. DO synchronize your breathing and your exercises. Always exhale on the exertion.

3. DON'T do any exercise that hurts. Progress doesn't mean pushing and straining during exercise. Pain is a warning that means *stop*. Listen to it. If an exercise produces pain, it may be that you are performing it incorrectly or that it is too difficult for your fitness level and should be attempted only after you can perform less demanding exercises easily. If pain does not stop or if it becomes more severe, seek medical help right away so that your physician can make a proper diagnosis and determine which exercises are inappropriate for you at this time.

4. DO move slowly and smoothly. DON'T do any fast or jerky movement, which might strain a muscle or a joint.

5. DO make sure you aren't tensing up one body part while you are exercising another.

6. DON'T "tighten your gluteals" as so many exercise books suggest. You are trying to undo muscular tightness. Use imagery and stretching to achieve a more desirable effect.

7. DON'T stretch your hamstrings if you have sciatic pain.

8. DON'T bend forward with your knees straight. Keep them "soft" and slightly bent.

9. DO place your hands under your buttocks when performing abdominal exercises while your legs are extended up toward the ceiling. This will prevent hyperextension (swayback) of the lower spine.

10. DON'T perform full sit-ups with your legs fully extended or with your knees bent. (Full sit-ups are those performed from the supine position all the way up to vertical.) When you do a full sit-up, the abdominal muscles are used only in the first thirty degrees of the exercise; the rest of the work to come up to a full vertical sit is done by the psoas, which is already shortened and tightened enough. Try a full sit-up and observe the point where your body makes a slight jerk or pull to come all the way up. That's the point where your abdominals stop doing the work of pulling you up and instead stabilize the pelvis in order for the psoas to complete the work of sitting up. The little "glitch" that you feel when you come up is when the muscle groups used to pull you up switch from the abdominals to the psoas.

11. NEVER DO straight-leg raises from the floor to the ceiling. This places too much strain on the lower back. Bent-knee leg raises allow the abdominals to contract more fully without help from the psoas (hip flexors) and won't cause additional tension in your lower back. And bent-knee curls or crunches will allow the abdominals to do their work in the thirty-degree radius without the aid of the psoas.

Ready for your workout? Let's go!

Weekly Workout Diary

SUNDAY   Type of Workout:
Duration:
Repetitions:
Comments:

MONDAY   Type of Workout:
Duration:
Repetitions:
Comments:

TUESDAY   Type of Workout:
Duration:
Repetitions:
Comments:

WEDNESDAY   Type of Workout:
Duration:
Repetitions:
Comments:

THURSDAY   Type of Workout:
Duration:
Repetitions:
Comments:

FRIDAY   Type of Workout:
Duration:
Repetitions:
Comments:

SATURDAY   Type of Workout:
Duration:
Repetitions:
Comments:

The Workouts

THE WARM-UP

A good warm-up is essential for safety and injury prevention. There are many ways to perform a good warm-up, provided that these five basic criteria are met:

1. Your breathing rate should increase to enable your respiratory system to meet the increased demand for oxygen.
2. Your heart rate should increase so that more oxygen-filled blood can be carried to the muscles.
3. After moving all the joints of the body, they should feel looser and less stiff.
4. There should be an increased blood flow to the muscles, making them more resilient and pliable as a result of the rise in temperature.
5. Your body should be able to respond more quickly to your commands, because the nerve impulses will travel faster through the warmed tissues.

The most effective movements for a warm-up involve sequences that require the muscles to contract and relax rhythmically. These movements should not be very vigorous, but they should involve all the joints. Stretching does not warm up the body properly, because stretching relaxes and lengthens the muscles and a warm-up should contract and move the muscles, literally warming you up.

The best way to start a warm-up is to lie supine on the floor. This enables you to warm the joints up before they have to bear the weight of the body. Your warm-up should be simple and gradually build in intensity, using energizing movements.

Lying on your back, relax and breathe deeply.

1. *Baby kicks*—Bend your knees to your chest and bounce your feet gently against your thighs.

2. *Shake it*—Shake your legs out. Shake your arms out. Shake your whole self out.

3. *Thigh circles*—With your hands on top of your knees, move your thighs in circles, working deep in the hip socket. Circle inwardly and outwardly. Keep the movements steady and continuous and in a moderately slow tempo.

4. *Double-knee spinal spiral*—With your arms extended sideways and resting on the floor, drop both knees to the right side and let them rest on the floor. Gently twist your upper body in the opposite direction.

5. *Arm circles*—Remain in the position above and circle your top arm first inwardly and then outwardly.

Repeat #4 and #5 on your left side.

6. *Leg cycles*—Place your hands under your pelvis and prop yourself up on your elbows. Cycle your legs forward for ten repetitions and then reverse direction and cycle backward for ten repetitions.

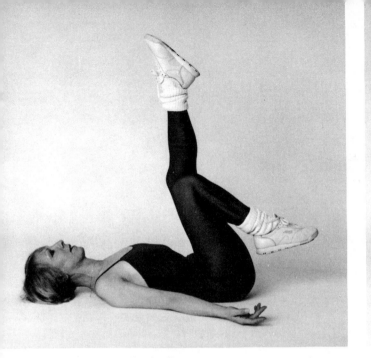

Figure 1. Baby kicks.

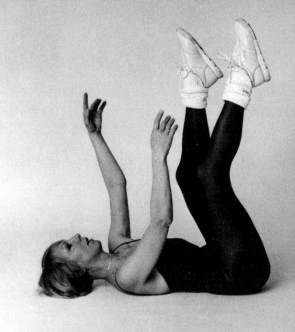

Figure 2. Shake it.

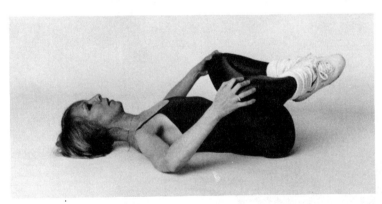

Figure 3. Thigh circles.

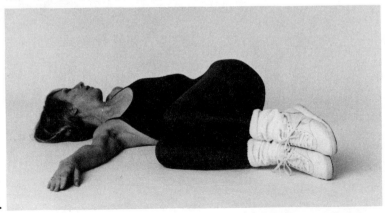

Figure 4. Double-knee spinal spiral.

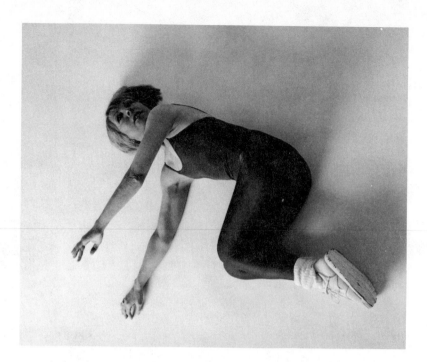

Figure 5. Arm circles.

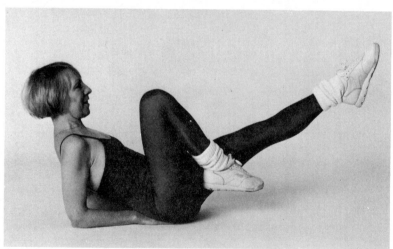

Figure 6. Leg cycles.

7. If you have time and want to continue the warm-up in the standing position. Move onto all fours and tread-walk in place.

8. Slowly rise to a standing position, keeping your spine rounded and knees bent.

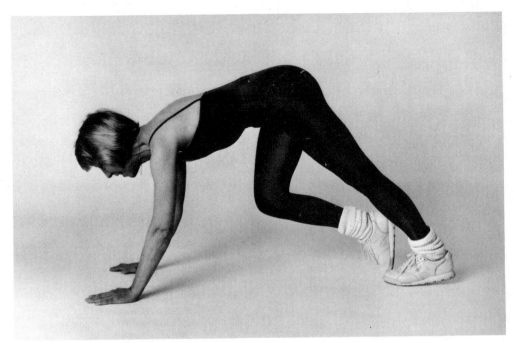

Figure 7. Tread-walk in place.

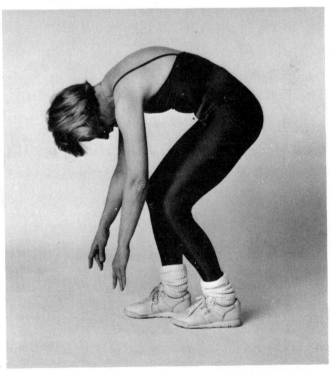

Figure 8. Round up the spine to vertical.

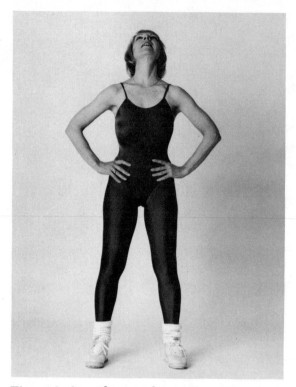

Figure 9. Stretch your chin to the ceiling.

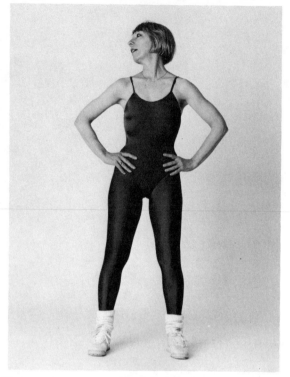

Figure 10. Rotate your head from right to left.

9. Gently drop your head forward and then stretch your chin to the ceiling.

10. Rotate your head from right to left and back again.

11. Tilt your head to your right shoulder as you raise the shoulder to meet it. Then tilt your head to your left shoulder.

12. Circle your arms up and over your head, forward and backward.

13. Reach out to the right side with your right arm, isolating your rib cage and holding your hips still. Repeat on the other side.

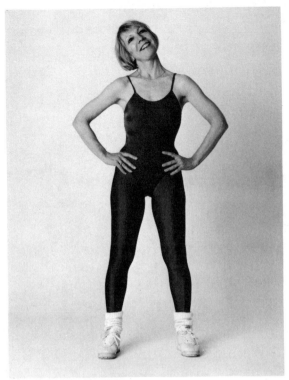

Figure 11. Tilt your head to your shoulder.

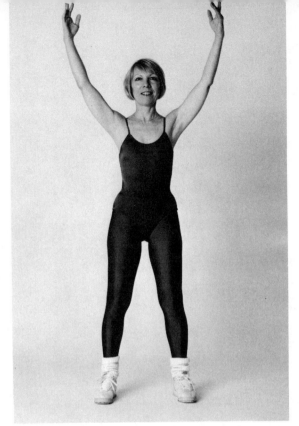

Figure 12. Circle the arms.

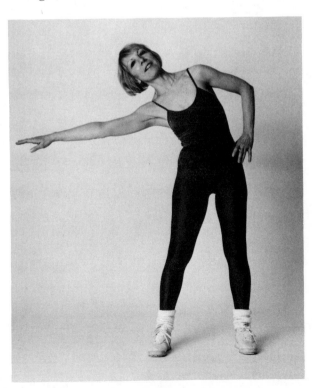

Figure 13. Reach out to the right side.

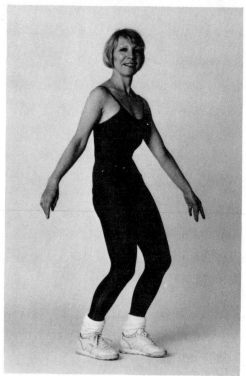

Figure 14. Move the pelvis forward and backward.

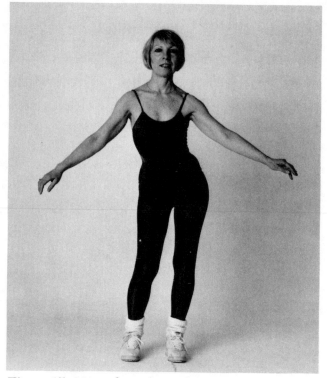

Figure 15. Move the pelvis side to side.

14. Move your pelvis forward and backward.

15. Move your pelvis side to side.

16. Bend the knees and shift left to right.

17. Keep shifting the weight from foot to foot and begin taking the feet off the floor.

18. Ease into a jog forward and backward.

Now you're warmed up and ready for the workout of your choice.

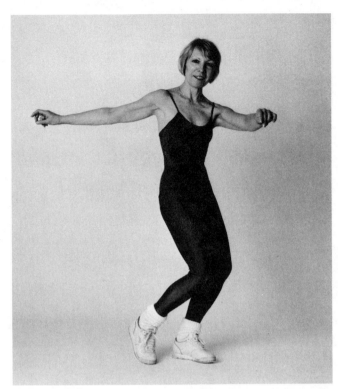

Figure 16. Bend the knees
and shift left to right.

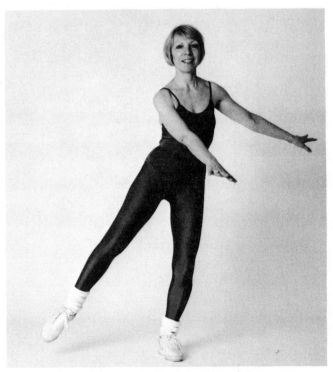

Figure 17. Shift the weight from foot to foot.

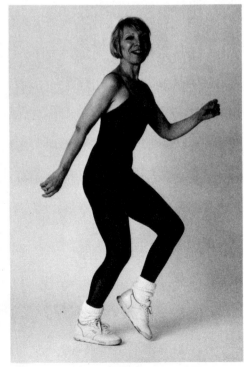

Figure 18. Ease into a jog.

Workout Sequence #1

1. *Double-Knee Hug*
2. *Double-Knee Spinal Spiral*
3. *Single-Knee Spiral*
4. *Hammock*
5. *Easy Hamstring Stretch*
6. *Psoas Release*
7. *Psoas Strengthener #1*
8. *Abdominals*
   A. *Pelvic Tilt*
   B. *Crunch with Knee Touch*
   C. *Diagonal Crunch with Knee Touch*
   D. *Toe Touch and Halfway Down*
   E. *Pop-up*
9. *Knee Drop*
10. *Psoas Side-Lying Stretch*
11. *Prone Single-Arm Raise*
12. *Prone Single-Leg Raise*
13. *Fold up and Unfold*
14. *Cheerleader Stretch*
15. *Knee Stretch*
16. *Painter's Stretch*

1. *Double-Knee Hug*

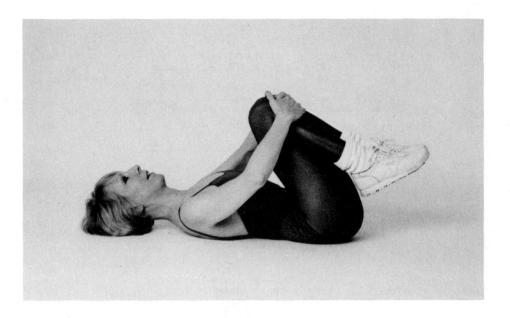

POSITION:

Lie supine, with your knees bent and feet flat on the floor.

ACTIVITY:

Tilt your pelvis, and bring both knees toward your chest without raising your head. Exhale and gently pull your knees as close to your chest as you can. Inhale, and then exhale as you lower your feet slowly to the floor.

IMAGE:

Imagine your pelvis sliding down on the floor toward where your feet would ordinarily be. Imagine that all of your vertebrae are moving in the opposite direction toward your head.

DURATION:

Thirty seconds.

2. *Double-Knee Spinal Spiral*

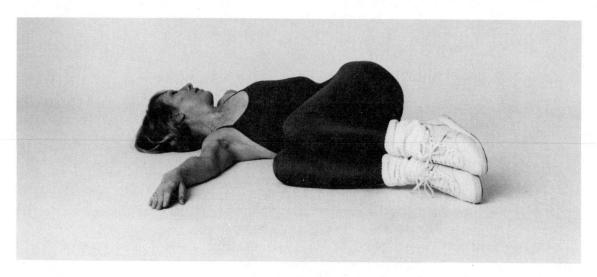

POSITION: Lie supine, with your knees bent and feet flat on the floor.

ACTIVITY: Inhale, and then exhale as you lift both knees to your chest. Inhale, and then exhale while you lower both knees to your right side, resting them on the floor. Gently twist your upper body and head to the opposite (left) side.

IMAGE: Imagine that your torso is like a spiral gently twisting your upper body opposite to your lower body.

DURATION: Thirty seconds.

Repeat on the other side.

3. Single-Knee Spiral

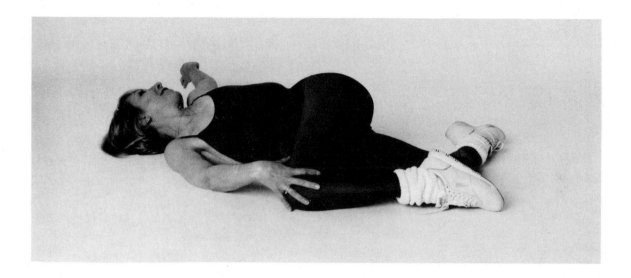

POSITION:	Lie supine, with your knees bent and feet flat on the floor.
ACTIVITY:	Raise your left knee to your chest; then drop it gently over to the right side on the floor. Turn your head to the left.
IMAGE:	Imagine that your body is like a towel gently twisting and spiraling the upper portion of your torso in opposition to the lower portion.
DURATION:	Thirty seconds.

Repeat with your right leg dropping to your left side.

4. Hammock

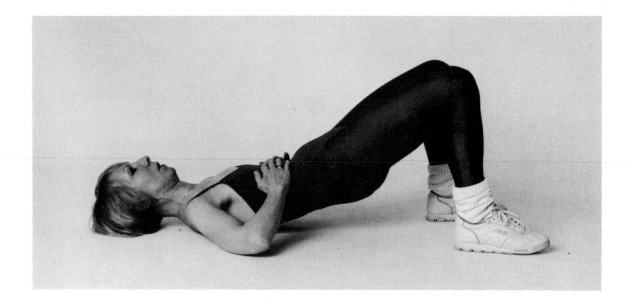

POSITION:	Lie supine, with your knees bent and feet flat on the floor.
ACTIVITY:	Inhale, and then exhale while slowly raising your hips up toward the ceiling. Inhale and then exhale as you slowly lower your hips back down to the floor.
IMAGE:	Imagine that the inhalation begins at your pelvis and travels up your back. See your back opening and widening out to the sides. The exhale passes your lips, your chin, your sternum, and your rib cage and drops down into your abdominals as you raise your hips upward. Use the same image for breathing as you lower the hips to the floor.
REPETITIONS:	Four.

This exercise is called the hammock because you should look as though you were being suspended from the ceiling by your knees with the rest of your spine sloping downward from that suspension. Do not push your ribs up to the ceiling. Instead, put your hands on your rib cage to encourage the ribs to drop down to the floor instead of pushing upward. Your spine should be round and long, not short and arched.

5. *Easy Hamstring Stretch*

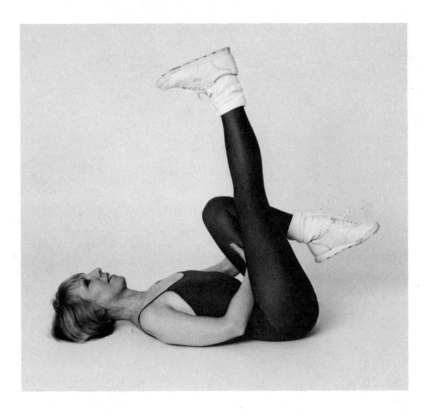

POSITION:	Lie supine, with both knees raised up to your chest. Hold onto your left thigh with both hands.
ACTIVITY:	Stretch your right leg up to the ceiling with the foot extended to the ceiling. Exhale as you flex the foot back to your face.
IMAGE:	Imagine that you have a dot placed on your right "sitz bone" (the two bones of the pelvis that you sit on) and another dot at the back of the heel. Connect the two dots with an imaginary straight line as you flex the heel up to the ceiling. Repeat with your left leg stretched up to the ceiling.
DURATION:	Fifteen seconds.

6. *Psoas Release*

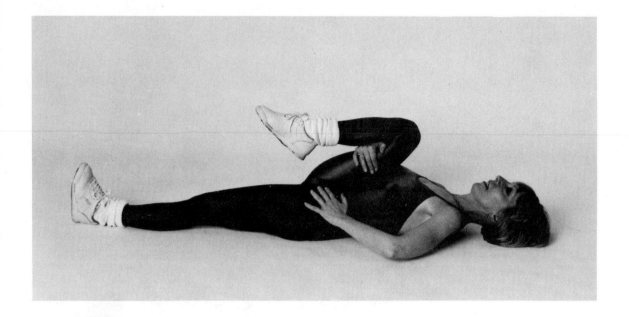

POSITION: Lie supine. Bend your right knee to your chest and lengthen your left leg along the floor.

ACTIVITY: Softly tug the right knee closer to your chest.

IMAGE: Breathing deeply, imagine that you have a water fountain spouting up through your left hip toward the ceiling. Imagine the water softly spraying around your hip joint and down your leg, allowing your leg to release.

DURATION: Thirty seconds.

Repeat with the other leg.

7. Psoas Strengthener #1

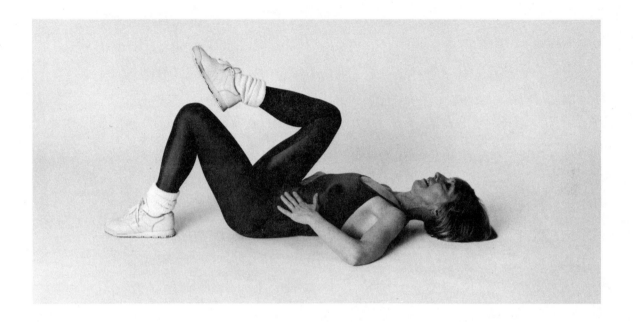

POSITION: Lie supine, with your knees bent and feet flat on floor.

ACTIVITY: Keep your right knee bent, and raise it to your chest while trying to keep your abdominal muscles soft. Slowly place the right foot back down on the floor and repeat with the left knee.

IMAGE: Imagine that your leg is very heavy as you draw it slowly upward to your chest.

REPETITIONS: Ten.

8. *Abdominals*

A. PELVIC TILT

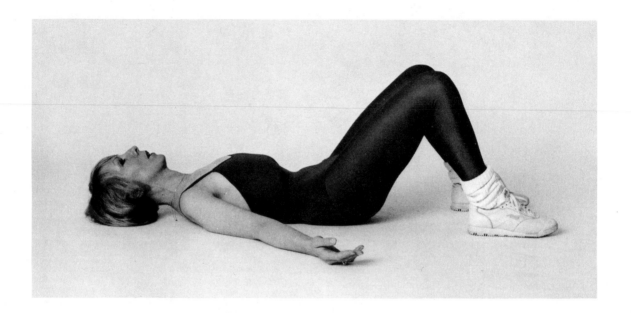

POSITION:	Lie supine, with your knees bent and feet flat on the floor.
ACTIVITY:	Inhale, and then exhale as you pull your abdomen in toward your spine while flattening the back against the floor.
IMAGE:	Imagine that your belly button is a vortex, where a swirling mass of water drains down to the floor.
REPETITIONS:	Ten.

B. CRUNCH WITH KNEE TOUCH

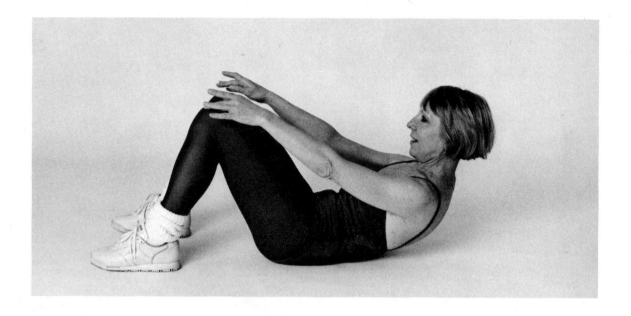

POSITION: Lie supine, with your knees bent and feet flat on floor.

ACTIVITY: Inhale, and then exhale as you tilt your pelvis to the floor and press your abdominals down, allowing your head and shoulders to come off the floor and reaching your arms toward your knees. Keep your neck and shoulders relaxed, and concentrate on pressing your belly button to your spine.

REPETITIONS: Ten to twenty.

C. DIAGONAL CRUNCH WITH KNEE TOUCH

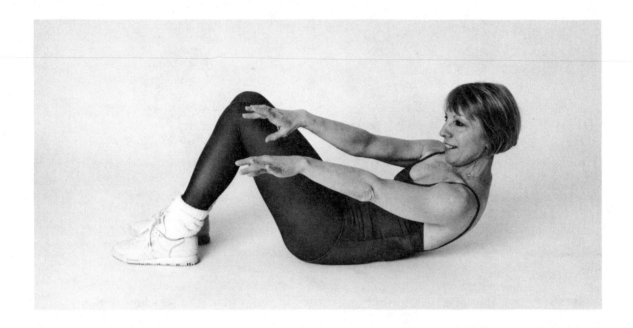

POSITION: Lie supine, with your knees bent and feet flat on floor.

ACTIVITY: Inhale, and then exhale as you tilt your pelvis to the floor and press your abdominals downward, allowing your head to come up. Reach your right hand toward your left knee. Keep your belly button pressed down to the floor.

REPETITIONS: Ten with the right hand reaching toward the left knee and ten with the left hand reaching toward the right knee.

D. TOE TOUCH AND HALFWAY DOWN

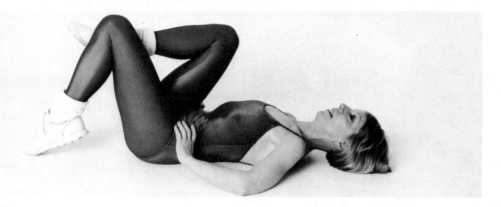

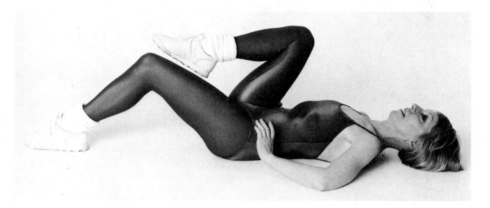

POSITION:	Lie supine, with your knees bent and raised up to your chest.
ACTIVITY 1:	Toe touch: Inhale, and then exhale while pressing your belly button down to the floor as you touch the tip of your left foot to the floor, keeping the right knee raised to the chest. Inhale, and then exhale as you raise your left foot back up to your chest. Repeat with the right foot.
REPETITIONS:	Alternating right and left, ten to twenty.
ACTIVITY 2:	Halfway down: With your right knee raised to the chest, place your left foot on the floor and slide it down only halfway to its full extension, so that your left knee remains bent. Alternate with your right leg.
REPETITIONS:	Ten to twenty.

E. POP-UP

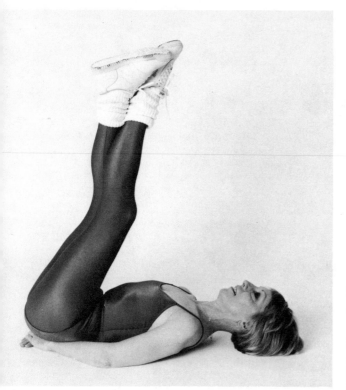

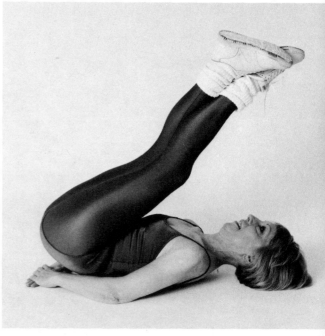

POSITION:	Lie supine, with your legs partially extended to the ceiling, and your feet crossed at the ankles. Place your hands under your pelvis.
ACTIVITY:	Inhale, and then exhale as you roll your legs toward your upper torso. Feel your lower back lengthen and stretch as you gently rock your pelvis down to the floor.
REPETITIONS:	Ten with your left ankle on top of the right, and ten with the right ankle on top of the left.

9. *Knee Drop*

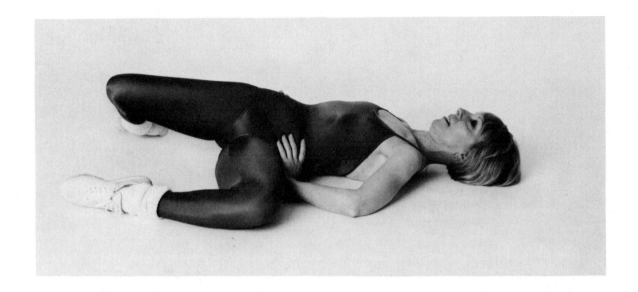

POSITION:	Lie supine, with your knees bent and feet flat on floor.
ACTIVITY:	Inhale, and then exhale while dropping both knees to the floor on the left side. The left leg will turn out and the right leg will turn in.
IMAGE:	See a rotating wheel on your right pelvic crest bone. It is rotating counterclockwise toward the floor. See an opposite line of energy going from the crest bone down along the thighbone toward the knee. (This image should help keep you from arching your lower back.)
DURATION:	Thirty seconds.
	Repeat with the other leg.

10. *Psoas Side-Lying Stretch*

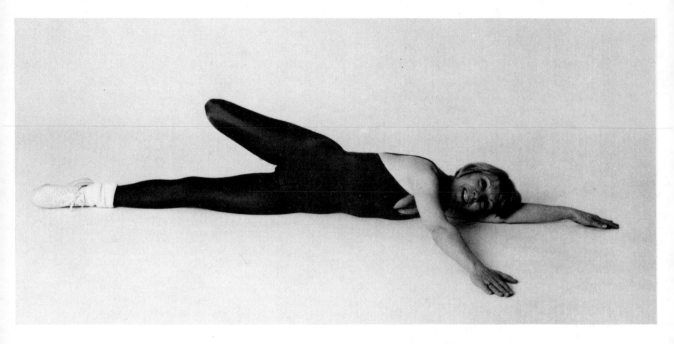

POSITION: Lie on your left side with your left leg straight and right knee bent behind you. Extend your left arm straight above your head.

ACTIVITY: Stretch your right leg behind you on a diagonal, and reach diagonally forward with your right arm.

IMAGE: As you are twisting your lower body in opposition to your upper body, imagine that you are creating an opening or a space in the front of your right hip socket.

DURATION: Thirty to sixty seconds.

Repeat with the other leg.

11. *Prone Single-Arm Raise*

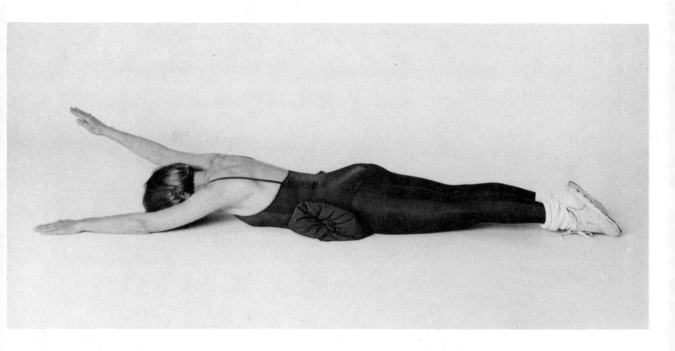

POSITION: Lie prone with a pillow under your hips.

ACTIVITY: Inhale, and then exhale as you raise your right arm as high as possible above your head, keeping your elbow straight. Relax the arm down. Repeat with your left arm. Don't arch your back.

REPETITIONS: Alternate ten times.

12. *Prone Single-Leg Raise*

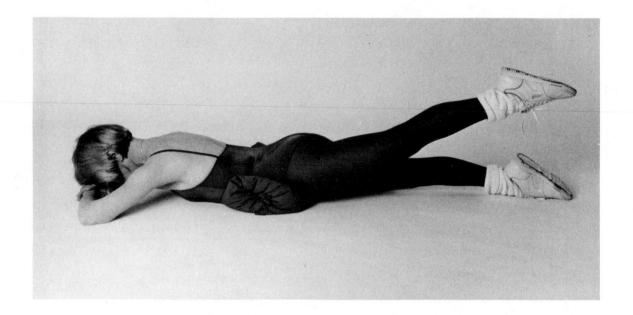

POSITION: Lie prone, with pillow under your hips, and rest your forehead on your hands.

ACTIVITY: Inhale, and then exhale as you raise your left leg with your knee straight. Relax your leg down. Don't arch your back. Repeat with your right leg.

REPETITIONS: Alternate ten times.

13. *Fold up and Unfold*

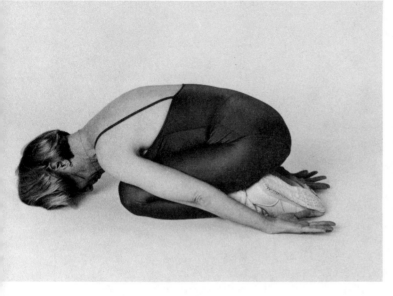
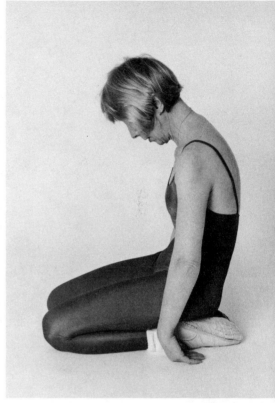

POSITION: On your knees with your forehead on the floor, fold up into a fetal position with your arms down along your sides.

ACTIVITY: Roll your spine up to sitting with your buttocks resting on your heels. Drop your head down and slowly roll your spine back down to the floor until you are back in the original fetal position.

IMAGE: Keep your thoughts focused on your vertebrae. As you round your spine up to the vertical position, imagine that you see an elevator that starts at the ground-floor level (your pelvis) and travels upward toward your head. On the descent, see the elevator start from the top floor and go down vertebra by vertebra until it reaches the ground level once again.

DURATION: Sixty seconds.

14. *Cheerleader Stretch*

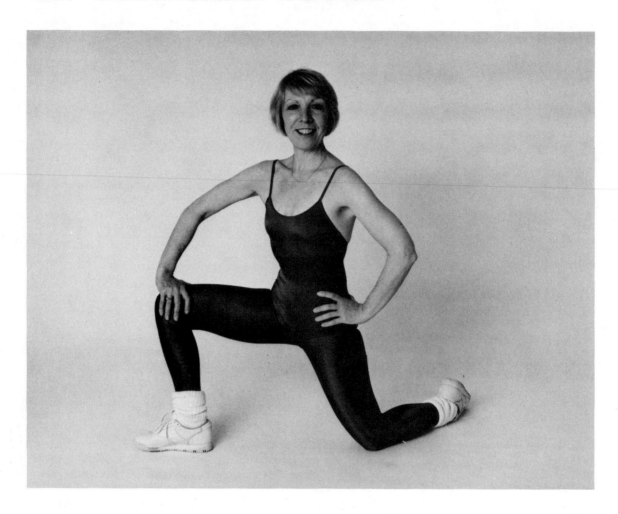

POSITION:	Kneel on your left knee with your right foot flat on the floor.
ACTIVITY:	Push gently and stretch your left hip forward. Place your right hand on your right knee for support.
IMAGE:	Breathe into your left hip and imagine it expanding and opening like a beam of light.
DURATION:	Thirty to sixty seconds.
	Repeat with the other leg.

15. *Knee Stretch*

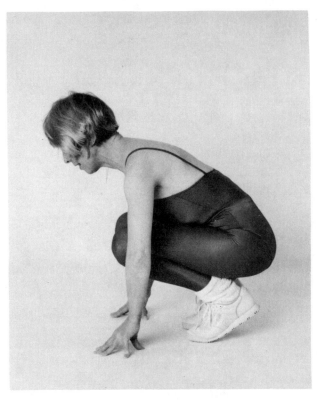 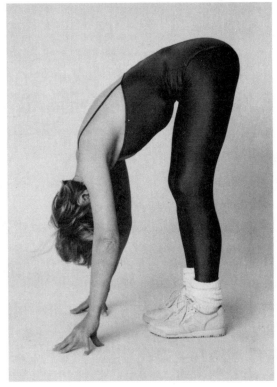

POSITION: Squat with your feet aligned under your hipbones and your hands on the floor.

ACTIVITY: Keeping your hands on the floor and your back round, slowly straighten your legs so that the buttocks stretch up toward the ceiling. Stay there and breathe. Do not extend your knees fully; keep them slightly bent. Slowly roll back down to the squatting position.

REPETITIONS: Four.

16. *Painter's Stretch*

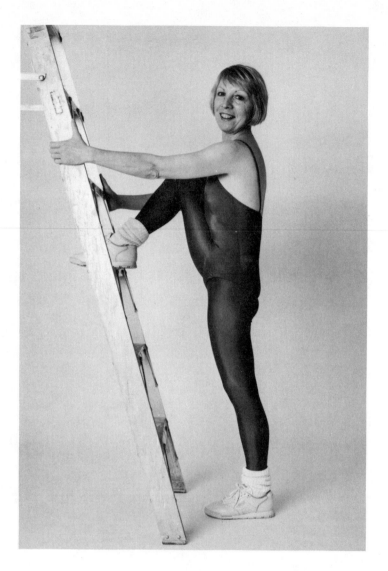

POSITION:	Stand on your left leg and bend your right knee and place your right foot on a desk, tabletop, ladder, or wall. Choose a height that you feel comfortable with; don't strain yourself.
ACTIVITY:	Push your left hip forward toward the desk.
IMAGE:	Imagine that a fountain of water sprays forward from your hip socket.
DURATION:	Thirty to sixty seconds.
	Repeat with the other leg.

PERSONAL PROGRESS CHART

Basic Back Workout—Level I   **EXERCISE #**

# Reps/Flexibility Level	Week #1	Week #2	Week #3	Week #4	Week #5	Week #6	Week #11	Week #12
1.								
2.								
3.								
4.								
5.								
6.								
7.								
8.								
9.								
10.								
11.								
12.								
13.								
14.								
15.								
16.								

Comments:

Workout Sequence #2

1. *Double-Knee Hug*
2. *Double-Knee Spinal Spiral*
3. *Single-Knee Spiral with Standing Leg Long*
4. *Hammock*
5. *Hamstring Stretch (with knee bent and foot flat)*
6. *Psoas Release with Head Lift*
7. *Psoas Strengthener #1*
8. *Abdominals*
    A. *Pelvic Tilt*
    B. *Crunch with Crossed Arms*
    C. *Diagonal Crunch with Crossed Arms*
    D. *Toe Touch, Halfway Down and Legs off the Floor*
    E. *Pop-up*
9. *Knee Drop*
10. *Psoas Side-Lying Stretch*
11. *Prone Double-Arm Raise*
12. *Prone Double-Leg Raise*
13. *Fold up and Unfold*
14. *Cheerleader Stretch with Elbows Forward*
15. *Knee Stretch*
16. *Painter's Stretch into Hamstring Stretch*

1. *Double-Knee Hug*

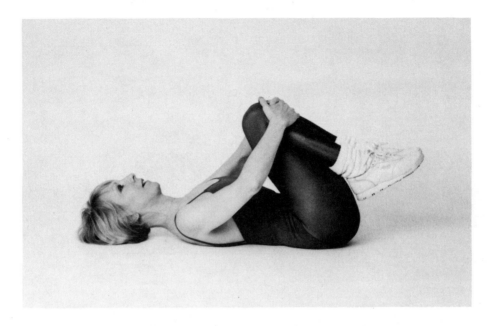

POSITION: Lie supine, with your knees bent and feet flat on the floor.

ACTIVITY: Tilt your pelvis, and bring both knees toward your chest without raising your head. Gently pull your knees as close to your chest as you can as you exhale. Inhale, and then exhale as you lower your feet slowly to the floor.

IMAGE: Imagine your pelvis sliding down on the floor toward where your feet would ordinarily be. Imagine that all of your vertebrae are moving in the opposite direction toward your head.

DURATION: Thirty seconds.

2. *Double-Knee Spinal Spiral*

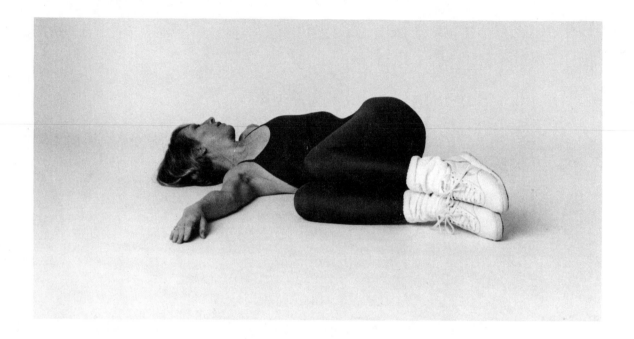

POSITION: Lie supine, with your knees bent and feet flat on the floor.

ACTIVITY: Inhale, and then exhale as you lift both knees to your chest.
Inhale, and then exhale as you lower both knees to your right
side, resting them on the floor. Gently twist your upper body
and head to the opposite (left) side.

IMAGE: Imagine that your torso is like a spiral gently twisting your
upper body opposite to your lower body.

DURATION: Thirty seconds.

Repeat on the other side.

3. Single-Knee Spiral with Standing Leg Long

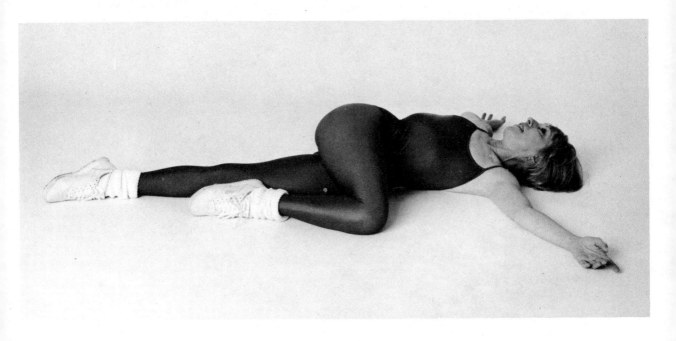

POSITION: Lie supine, with your knees bent and feet flat on the floor.

ACTIVITY: Raise your right knee to your chest. Stretch your left leg long along the floor. Drop your right knee over to the left side on the floor. Turn your head to the right.

IMAGE: Imagine that your body is like a towel gently twisting and spiraling the upper portion of your torso in opposition to the lower portion.

DURATION: Thirty seconds.

Repeat with your left knee dropping over to the right side on the floor.

4. *Hammock*

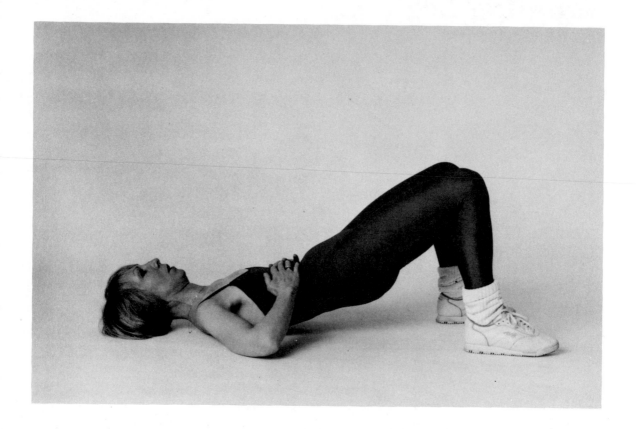

POSITION:	Lie supine, with your knees bent and feet flat on floor.
ACTIVITY:	Inhale, and then exhale while slowly raising your hips up toward the ceiling. Inhale and then exhale slowly as you lower your hips back down to the floor.
IMAGE:	Imagine that the inhalation begins at your pelvis and travels up your back. See your back opening and widening out to the sides. The exhale passes your lips, your chin, your sternum, and your rib cage and drops down into your abdominals as you raise your hips upward. Use the same image for breathing as you lower the hips to the floor.
REPETITIONS:	Four.

5. *Hamstring Stretch*

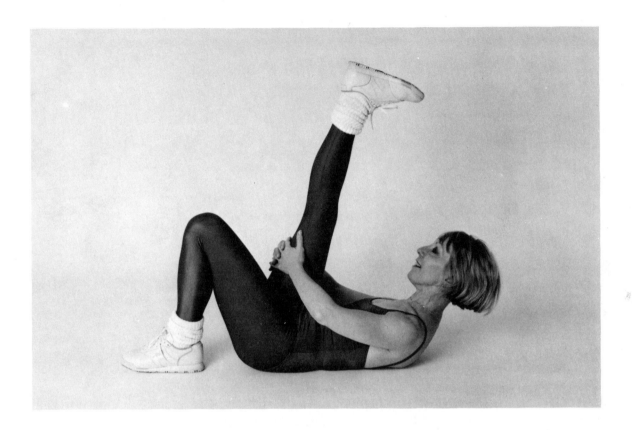

POSITION:	Lie supine, with your knees bent and your feet flat on floor.
ACTIVITY:	Keeping your left leg bent and the left foot flat on the floor, raise your right knee to your chest while holding onto the right thigh. Stretch your right leg to the ceiling with the right foot pointed. Breathe in, and lift your head to your extended leg as you exhale. Repeat the exercise with the right foot flexed.
IMAGE:	Image a dot at the right "sitz bone" and a dot at the back of the right heel. Connect the two dots with an imaginary straight line.
DURATION:	Thirty seconds.
	Repeat the exercise with your left leg.

6. *Psoas Release with Head Lift*

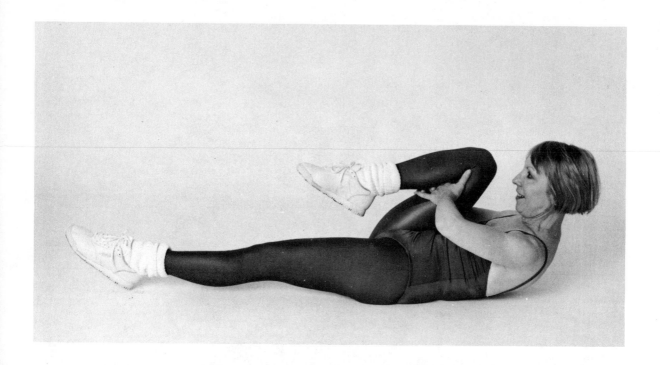

POSITION: Lie supine. Bend your right knee to your chest and lengthen your left leg along the floor.

ACTIVITY: Softly tug your right knee closer to your chest. Inhale, and then exhale as you raise your head to your knee.

IMAGE: Breathe deeply and imagine that you have a water fountain spouting up through your hip toward the ceiling. Imagine the water softly spraying around your hip joint and down your leg, allowing your leg to release.

DURATION: Thirty to sixty seconds.

Repeat with the other leg.

7. *Psoas Strengthener #1*

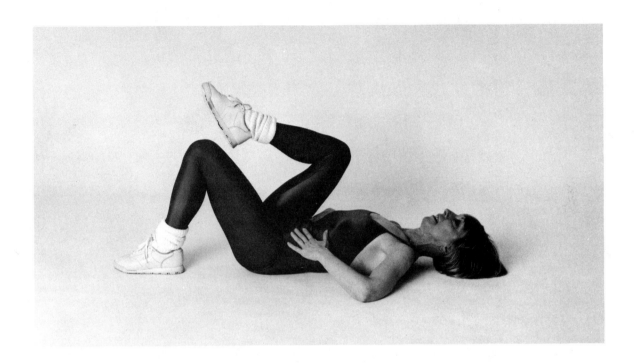

POSITION:	Lie supine, with your knees bent and feet flat on floor.
ACTIVITY:	Keep your right knee bent, and raise it to your chest while trying to keep your abdominal muscles soft. Slowly place the right foot back down on the floor and repeat with the left knee.
IMAGE:	Imagine that your leg is very heavy as you draw it slowly upward to your chest.
REPETITIONS:	Ten.

8. *Abdominals*

A. PELVIC TILT

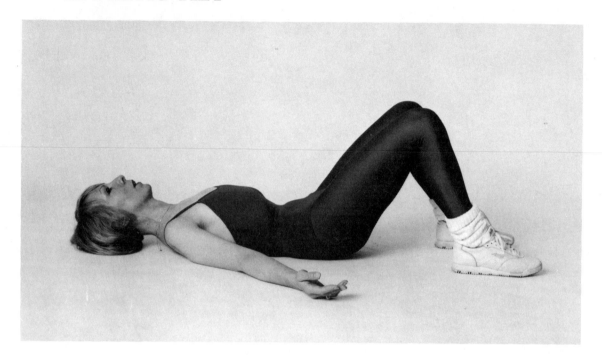

POSITION: Lie supine, with your knees bent and feet flat on the floor.

ACTIVITY: Inhale, and then exhale as you pull your abdomen in toward your spine while flattening the back against the floor.

IMAGE: Imagine that your belly button is a vortex, where a swirling mass of water drains down to the floor.

REPETITIONS: Ten.

B. CRUNCH WITH CROSSED ARMS

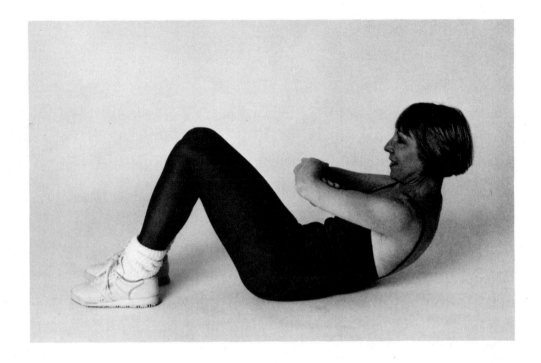

POSITION: Lie supine, with your knees bent and your feet flat on the floor.

ACTIVITY: Inhale, and then exhale as you tilt your pelvis down and press your abdominals to the floor, allowing your head and shoulders to come off the floor. Cross your arms in front of your chest with each hand grasping the opposite elbow. Concentrate on pressing your belly button to the ground.

REPETITIONS: Ten to twenty.

C. DIAGONAL CRUNCH WITH CROSSED ARMS

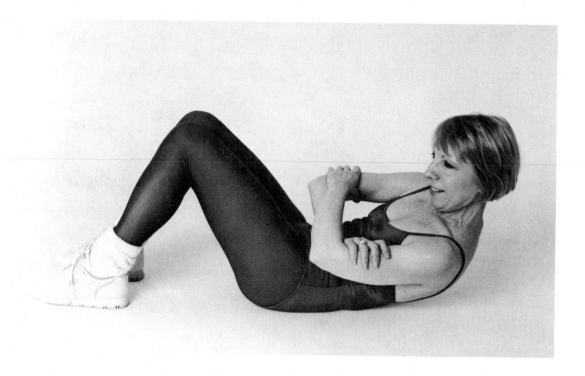

POSITION: Lie supine, with your knees bent and your feet flat on the floor.

ACTIVITY: Inhale, and then exhale as you tilt your pelvis to the floor. Press your abdominals downward, allowing your head to come up and your right shoulder to reach toward your left knee with your arms crossed in front of your chest. Keep your belly button pressed to the floor.

REPETITIONS: Ten with right diagonal twist; ten with left diagonal twist.

D. TOE TOUCH, HALFWAY DOWN AND LEGS OFF THE FLOOR

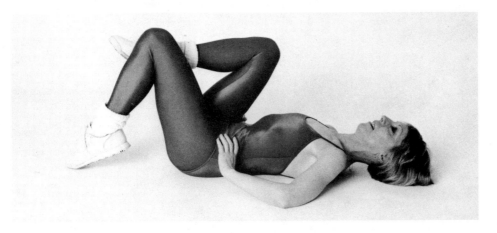

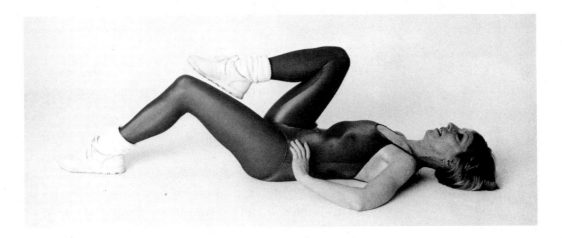

POSITION: Lie supine, with your knees bent and raised up to your chest.

ACTIVITY 1: Toe touch: Inhale, and then exhale while pressing your belly button down to the floor as you touch the tip of the left foot to the floor, keeping the right knee raised to the chest. Inhale, and then exhale as you raise your left foot back to your chest. Repeat with your right foot.

ACTIVITY 2: Halfway down: Keeping your right knee raised to your chest, slide your left foot along the floor only halfway down so that the knee remains bent. Alternate with your right leg.

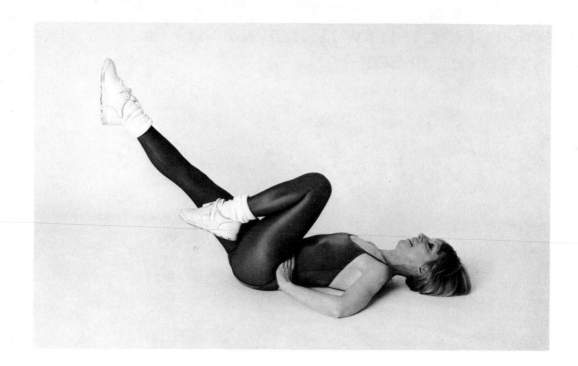

ACTIVITY 3: Off the floor: Continue the movement in Activity #2, but this time extend the right leg fully, keeping it 12 inches above the floor. Alternate with the left leg.

NOTE: If you cannot keep your lower back pressed down to the floor as you extend the legs forward, do not do this exercise until you can do so. If your abdominal muscles are weak, the weight of your legs going forward will pull the lower back off the floor, arching it and causing strain. Stop doing this section of the exercse until you are strong enough to keep the abdominals pressed to the floor.

REPETITIONS: Ten to twenty.

E. POP-UP

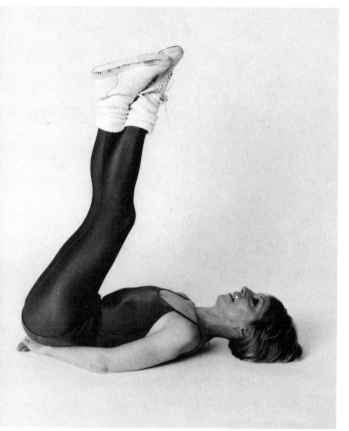

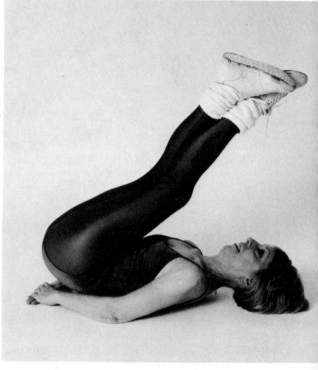

POSITION:	Lie supine, with your legs partially extended to the ceiling and your feet crossed at the ankles. Place your hands under your pelvis.
ACTIVITY:	Inhale, and then exhale and roll your legs toward your upper torso. Feel your lower back lengthen and stretch as you gently rock your pelvis down to the floor.
REPETITIONS:	Ten with your left ankle on top of the right, and ten with the right ankle on top of the left.

9. Knee Drop

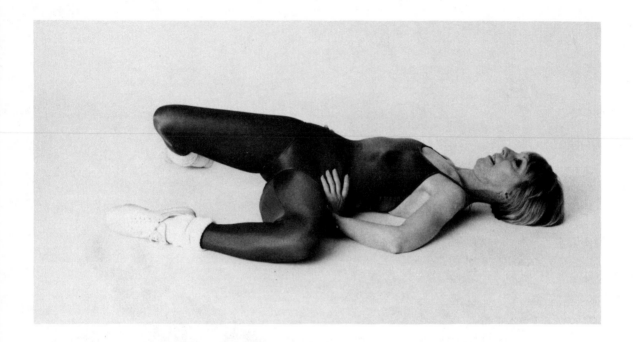

POSITION: Lie supine, with your knees bent and feet flat on the floor.

ACTIVITY: Inhale, and then exhale while dropping both knees to the floor on the left side. The left leg will turn out, and the right leg will turn in.

IMAGE: See a rotating wheel on your right pelvic crest bone. It is rotating counterclockwise toward the floor. See an opposite line of energy going from the crest bone down along the thighbone toward the knee. (This image should help to keep you from arching your lower back.)

DURATION: Thirty seconds.

Repeat with the other leg.

10. *Psoas Side-Lying Stretch*

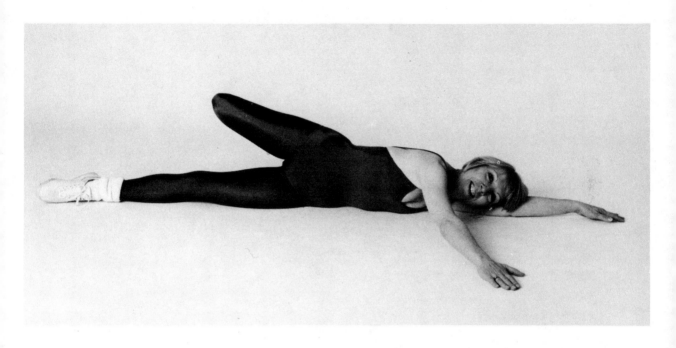

POSITION: Lie on your left side with your left leg straight and right knee bent behind you. Extend your left arm straight above your head.

ACTIVITY: Stretch your right leg behind you on a diagonal, and reach diagonally forward with your right arm.

IMAGE: As you are twisting your lower body in opposition to your upper body, imagine that you are creating an opening or a space in the front of your right hip socket.

DURATION: Thirty to sixty seconds.

Repeat with the other leg.

11. *Prone Double-Arm Raise*

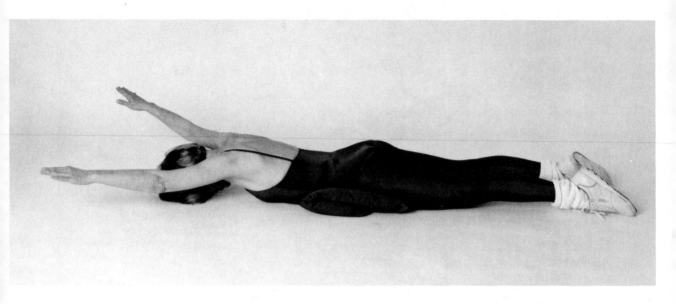

POSITION: Lie prone, with a pillow under your hips. Extend your arms diagonally overhead.

ACTIVITY: Inhale, and then exhale as you raise both arms up as high as possible, keeping your elbows straight. Relax down to the floor. Don't arch your back.

REPETITIONS: Ten.

12. *Prone Double-Leg Raise*

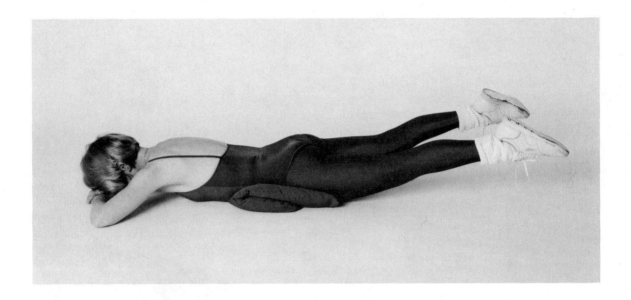

POSITION:	Lie prone, with a pillow under your hips. Rest your forehead on your hands. Extend your legs in a small V-position.
ACTIVITY:	Inhale, and then exhale as you raise both legs simultaneously as far off the floor as you are able. Lower your legs back down to the floor. Don't arch your back.
REPETITIONS:	Ten.

13. *Fold up and Unfold*

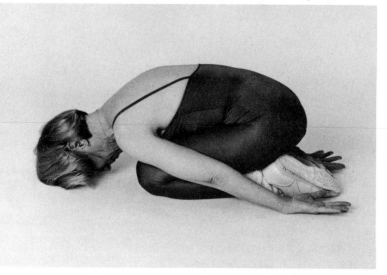
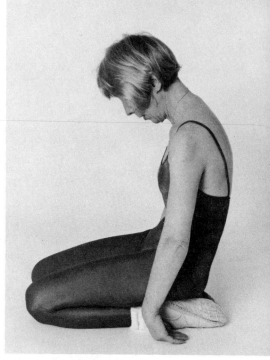

POSITION:	On your knees with your forehead on the floor, fold up into a fetal position with your arms down along your sides.
ACTIVITY:	Roll your spine up to sitting with your buttocks resting on your heels. Drop your head down and slowly roll your spine back down to the floor until you are back in the original fetal position.
IMAGE:	Keep your thoughts focused on your vertebrae. As you round your spine up to the vertical position, imagine that you see an elevator that starts at the ground-floor level (your pelvis) and travels upward toward your head. On the descent, see the elevator start from the top floor and go down vertebra by vertebra until it reaches the ground level once again.
DURATION:	Sixty seconds.

14. *Cheerleader Stretch with Elbows Forward*

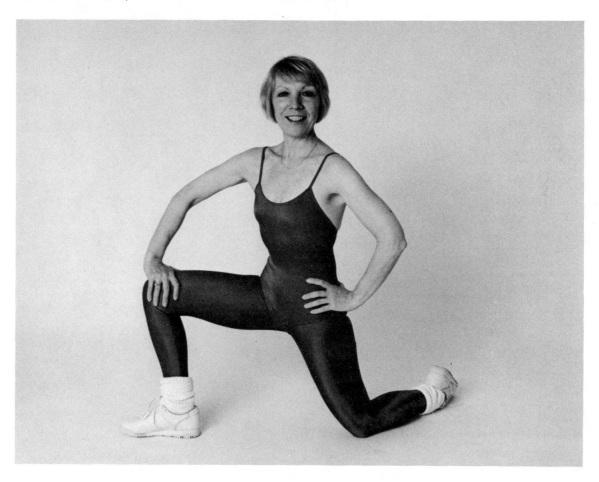

POSITION:	Kneel on your left knee with your right foot flat on the floor.
ACTIVITY:	Push gently and stretch your left hip forward, with your right hand on your right knee for support. Then place both elbows on your right knee and lean forward.
IMAGE:	Breathe into your left hip and imagine it expanding and opening like a beam of light.
DURATION:	Thirty to sixty seconds.
	Repeat with the other leg.

15. *Knee Stretch*

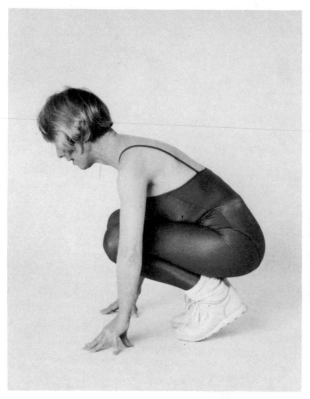 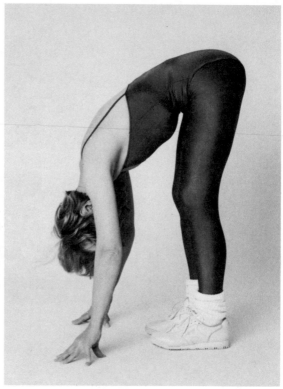

POSITION: Squat with your feet aligned under your hipbones and your hands on the floor.

ACTIVITY: Keeping your hands on the floor and your back round, slowly straighten your legs so that the buttocks stretch up toward the ceiling. Stay there and breathe. Do not extend your knees fully; keep them slightly bent. Slowly roll back down to the squatting position.

REPETITIONS: Four.

16. *Painter's Stretch into Hamstring Stretch*

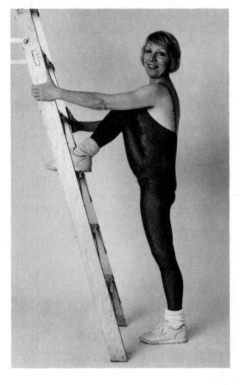 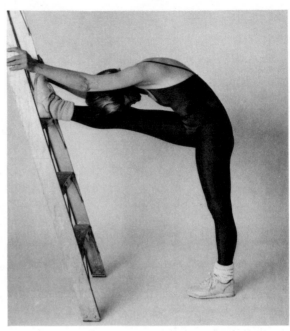

POSITION:	Stand on your left leg. Bend your right knee and place your right foot on a desk, tabletop, or ladder at a comfortable height.
ACTIVITY 1:	Push your left hip forward toward the desk.
IMAGE:	See a beam of light being projected forward from your left hip joint.
DURATION:	Thirty seconds.
ACTIVITY 2:	Hamstring stretch: Stretch your right leg forward on top of the desk. Inhale, and then exhale as you drop your head down toward your right knee.
IMAGE:	As you breathe, feel the weight of the head, neck, and shoulders pull the spine forward and down to your knee, like the bough of a tree being weighted down with heavy snow.
DURATION:	Thirty seconds.
	Repeat with the other leg.

PERSONAL PROGRESS CHART

Basic Back Workout—Level II   **EXERCISE #**

# Reps/Flexibility Level	Week #1	Week #2	Week #3	Week #4	Week #5	Week #6	Week #11	Week #12
1.								
2.								
3.								
4.								
5.								
6.								
7.								
8.								
9.								
10.								
11.								
12.								
13.								
14.								
15.								
16.								

Comments:

Workout Sequence #3

1. *Double-Knee Hug with Knee Kiss*
2. *Double-Knee Spiral with Both Legs Stretched*
3. *Single-Knee Spiral with Top Leg Stretched*
4. *Hammock*
5. *Drop, Swing, Flex with Hamstring Stretch*
6. *Psoas Release with Head Lift*
7. *Psoas Strengthener #2*
8. *Abdominals*
   A. *Pelvic Tilt*
   B. *Crunch with Hands Clasped Behind Head*
   C. *Diagonal Crunch with Hands Clasped Behind Head*
   D. *Toe Touch, Halfway Down and Legs off Floor with Head up*
   E. *Crunch with Legs up*
   F. *Pop-up*
9. *Knee Drop*
10. *Psoas Stretch from All Fours to Floor*
11. *Single Arm and Leg Raise*
12. *Chin and Chest Raise*
13. *Fold up into Hip Stretch*
14. *Psoas Racer's Stretch*
15. *Knee Stretch, Hamstring Stretch, and Back Strengthener*
16. *Painter's Stretch into Hamstring Stretch*
17. *Psoas Bow Stretch*

1. Double-Knee Hug with Knee Kiss

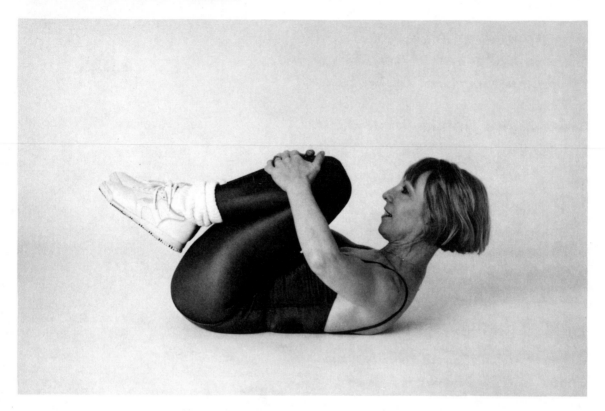

POSITION:	Lie supine, with your knees bent and your feet flat on the floor.
ACTIVITY:	Tilt your pelvis, and bring both knees toward your chest. Inhale and then exhale and gently pull your knees as close to your chest as you can. Inhale, and then exhale as you raise your head and shoulders off the floor. Bring your head and knees as close together as possible.
IMAGE:	Imagine that you are creating space and distance between each vertebra as you stretch forward to kiss your knees.
DURATION:	Thirty seconds.

2. Double-Knee Spiral with Both Legs Stretched

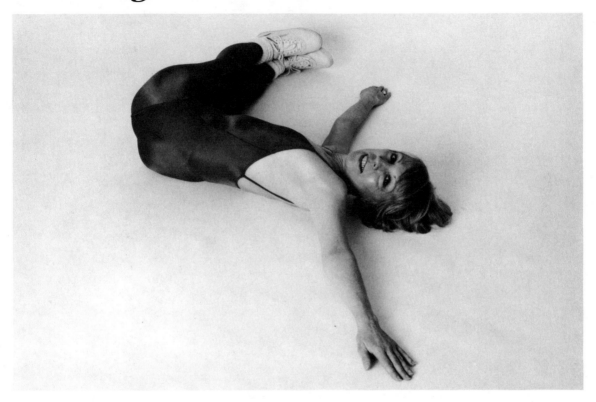

POSITION: Lie supine, with your knees bent and your feet flat on the floor. Stretch your arms out from your shoulders.

ACTIVITY: Inhale, and then exhale as you raise both knees to your chest. Inhale, and then exhale as you lower both knees to your right side, resting them on the floor. Twist your head to your left side. Inhale, and then exhale as you stretch both legs out straight to your right hand. Inhale, and then exhale and bend your knees as you return to your back.

IMAGE: See the spiraling energy of your spine continue out through both legs.

DURATION: Thirty to sixty seconds.

Repeat on the other side.

3. Single-Knee Spiral
with Top Leg Stretched

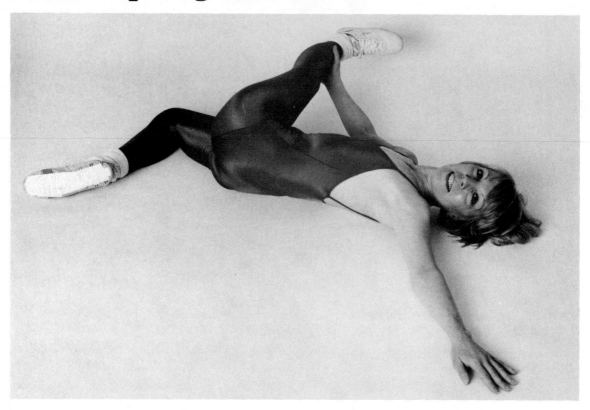

POSITION: Lie supine, with your knees bent, feet flat on the floor, and arms outstretched from your shoulders.

ACTIVITY: Inhale, and then exhale as you raise your left knee to your chest. Drop your left knee over to the right side on the floor. Turn your head to the left. Inhale, and then exhale as you stretch your left leg out straight to your right hand.

IMAGE: Imagine that you are sending a beam of light from the buttocks, along the back of the leg, and out from the foot into space.

DURATION: Thirty to sixty seconds.

Repeat with the other leg.

4. *Hammock*

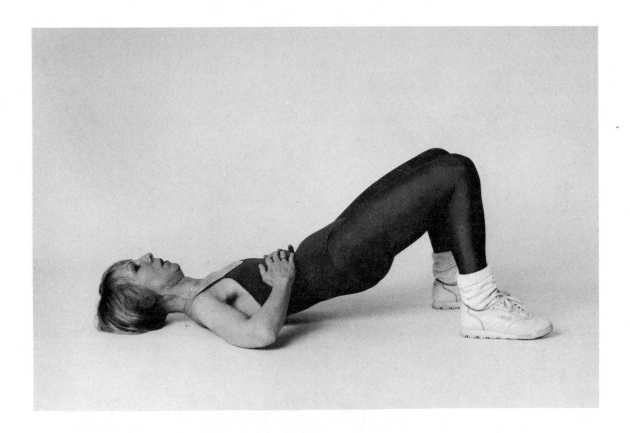

POSITION:	Lie supine, with your knees bent and feet flat on the floor.
ACTIVITY:	Inhale, and then exhale slowly while raising your hips up toward the ceiling. Inhale and then exhale while slowly lowering your hips back down to the floor.
IMAGE:	Imagine that the inhalation begins at your pelvis and travels up your back. See your back opening and widening out to the sides. The exhale passes your lips, your chin, your sternum, and your rib cage and drops down into your abdominals as you raise your hips upward. Use the same image for breathing as you lower the hips to the floor.
REPETITIONS:	Four.

5. Drop, Swing, Flex with Hamstring Stretch

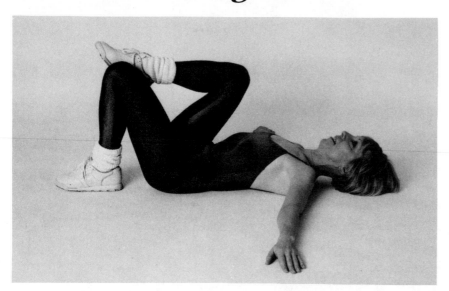

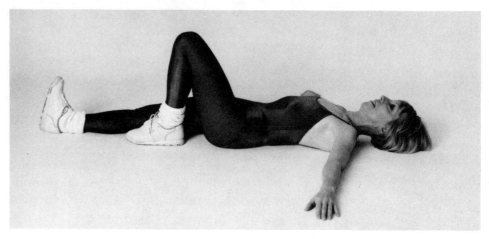

POSITION:	Lie supine, with your knees bent and feet flat on the floor.
ACTIVITY 1:	Raise your right knee to your chest, and then drop your right foot onto the floor and let it slide downward. When the right leg is almost completely extended, flex your right foot and swing the leg up to the ceiling. Then bend the right knee back to your chest.

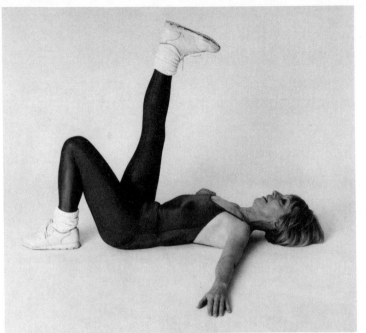

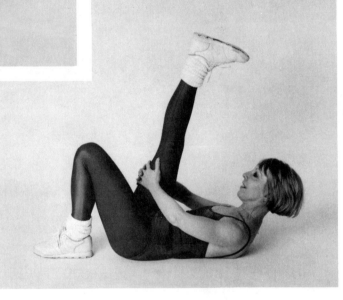

IMAGE:	For drop, swing, flex, visualize the movements of the ankle, knee, and hip joints as fluid as those of a marionette.
ACTIVITY 2:	Hamstring stretch: Bend your right knee up to your chest. Hold onto your right thigh with both hands. Inhale, and then exhale as you stretch your right leg to the ceiling. Flex your right foot and hold for thirty seconds. Inhale, and then exhale as you raise your head up to the right leg.
REPETITIONS:	Ten.
	Repeat with the other leg.

6. *Psoas Release with Head Lift*

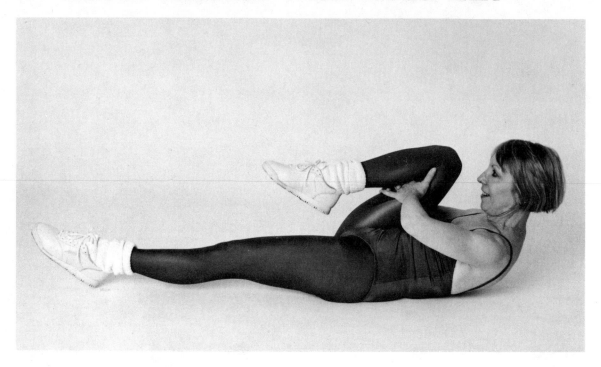

POSITION: Lie supine. Bend your right knee to your chest and lengthen your left leg along the floor.

ACTIVITY: Softly tug your right knee closer to your chest. Inhale, and then exhale as you raise your head to your knee.

IMAGE: Breathe deeply and imagine that you have a water fountain spouting up through your left hip toward the ceiling. Imagine the water softly spraying around your hip joint and down your leg, allowing your leg to release.

DURATION: Thirty to sixty seconds.

Repeat with the other leg.

7. Psoas Strengthener #2

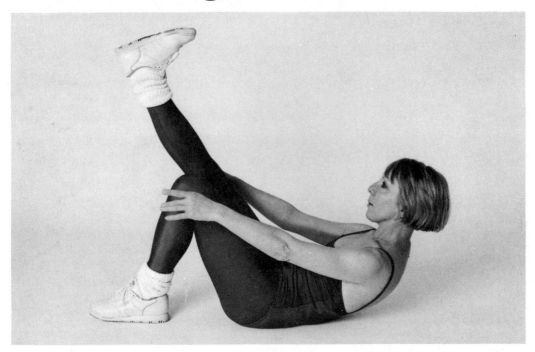

Single straight-leg raises:

POSITION:
Lie supine, with your knees bent and your feet flat on the floor.

ACTIVITY:
Tilt your pelvis and keep your left leg bent at both the hip and the knee. Slowly stretch the right leg and raise it to the same level as the bent knee so that both thighs are parallel. Flex the right foot and keep the right leg there and inhale. Exhale as you raise your head.

IMAGE:
Imagine that your belly button is the central vortex through which energy swirls downward to the floor as the extended leg arcs upward to the opposite leg.

REPETITIONS:
Ten.

Repeat with the other leg.

NOTE:
As your strength improves, you can try adding ankle weights to the extended leg. Start with one-pound weights and slowly work your way up to five-pound weights.

8. *Abdominals*

A. PELVIC TILT

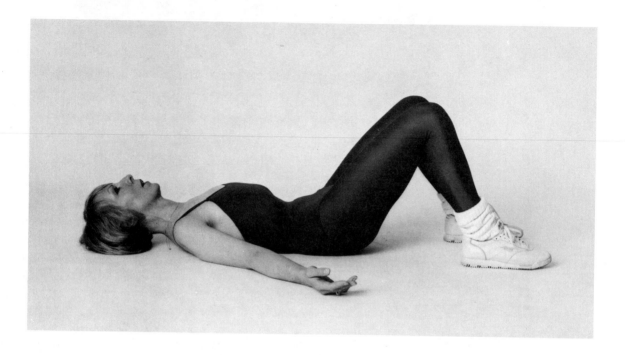

POSITION:	Lie supine, with your knees bent and feet flat on the floor.
ACTIVITY:	Inhale, and then exhale as you pull your abdomen in toward your spine while flattening the back against the floor.
IMAGE:	Imagine that your belly button is a vortex, where a swirling mass of water drains down to the floor.
REPETITIONS:	Ten.

B. CRUNCH WITH HANDS CLASPED BEHIND HEAD

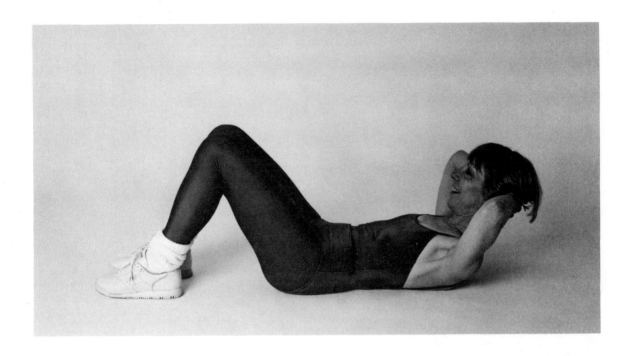

POSITION:	Lie supine, with your knees bent and your feet flat on the floor.
ACTIVITY:	Inhale, and then exhale as you tilt your pelvis to the floor and press your abdominals to the floor. Raise your head and shoulders off the floor with your hands clasped behind your head. Keep your neck and shoulders relaxed, and be sure to keep your belly button pressed down toward the floor.
REPETITIONS:	Ten to twenty.
NOTE:	To make this exercise harder, keep your elbows spread wide and kept back behind your ears.

C. DIAGONAL CRUNCH WITH HANDS CLASPED BEHIND HEAD

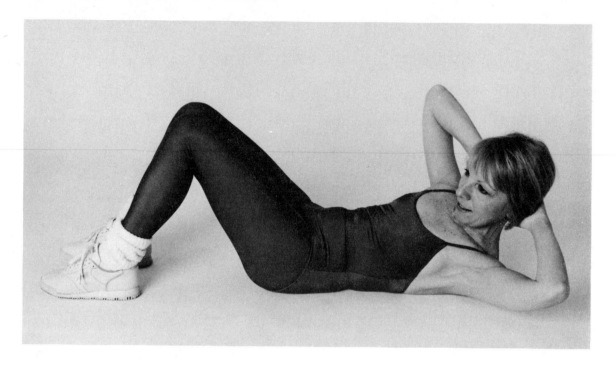

POSITION:	Lie supine, with your knees bent and your feet flat on the floor.
ACTIVITY:	Inhale, and then exhale as you tilt your pelvis to the floor, pressing your abdominals downward. Raise your head up, and twist your right shoulder toward your left knee with your hands clasped behind your head. Keep your belly button pressed to the floor.
REPETITIONS:	Ten with a right twist; ten with a left twist.
NOTE:	To make this exercise harder, keep your elbows wide apart and back behind your ears.

D. TOE TOUCH, HALFWAY DOWN AND LEGS OFF FLOOR WITH HEAD UP

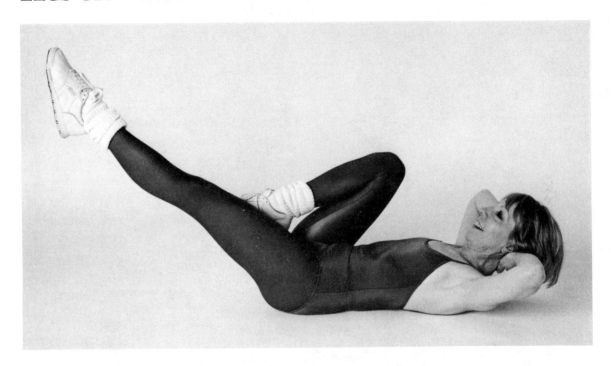

POSITION:	Lie supine, with your knees bent and raised up to your chest.
ACTIVITY:	Repeat the activity for toe touch, halfway down, and legs off the floor. Repeat the activity of extending your legs downward and off the floor with your head and shoulders off the floor and your hands clasped behind your head.
REPETITIONS:	Ten to twenty.

E. CRUNCH WITH LEGS UP

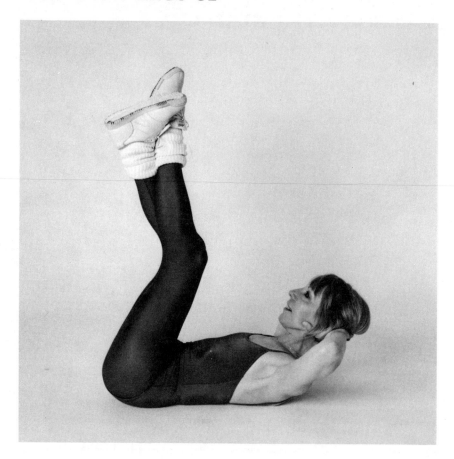

POSITION:

Lie supine, with your legs partially extended to the ceiling and your feet crossed at your ankles. Clasp your hands behind your head.

ACTIVITY:

Inhale, and then exhale as you raise your head, neck, and shoulders off the floor toward your legs. Keep your belly button pressed down to the floor.

REPETITIONS:

Ten to twenty.

F. POP-UP

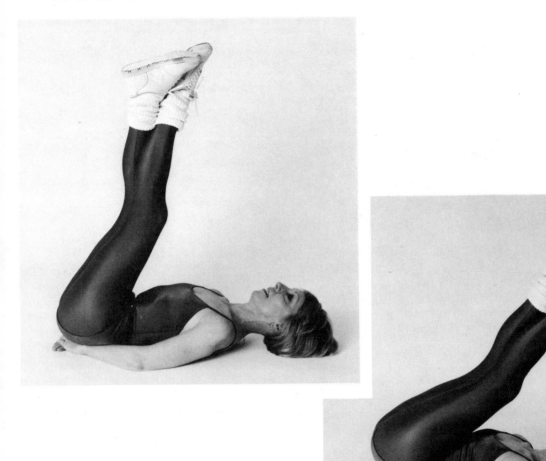

POSITION: Lie supine, with your legs partially extended to the ceiling and your feet crossed at the ankles. Place your hands under your pelvis.

ACTIVITY: Inhale, and then exhale as you roll your legs toward your upper torso. Feel your lower back lengthen and stretch as you gently rock your pelvis down to the floor.

REPETITIONS: Ten to twenty.

9. *Knee Drop*

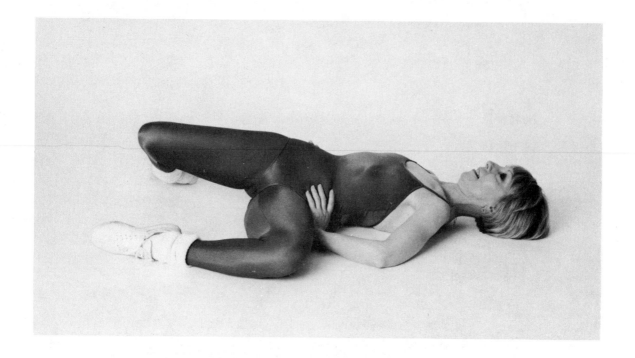

POSITION: Lie supine, with your knees bent and feet flat on the floor.

ACTIVITY: Inhale, and then exhale while dropping both knees to the floor on the left side. The left leg will turn out, and the right leg will turn in.

IMAGE: See a rotating wheel on your right pelvic crest bone. It is rotating counterclockwise toward the floor. See an opposite line of energy going from the crest bone down along the thighbone toward the knee. (This image should help to keep you from arching your lower back.)

DURATION: Thirty seconds.

Repeat with the other leg.

10. *Psoas Stretch from All Fours to Floor*

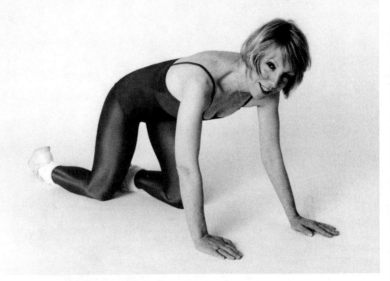

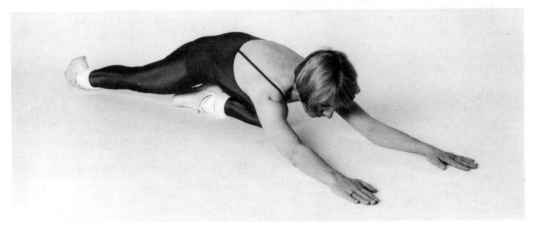

POSITION:	Kneel on your hands and knees.
ACTIVITY:	Slide your right leg long behind you until your head reaches the floor and your arms are stretched forward.
IMAGE:	Imagine that you are hanging from your arms and that your leg is dropping and lengthening downward.
DURATION:	Thirty to sixty seconds.
	Repeat with the other leg.

11. *Single Arm and Leg Raise*

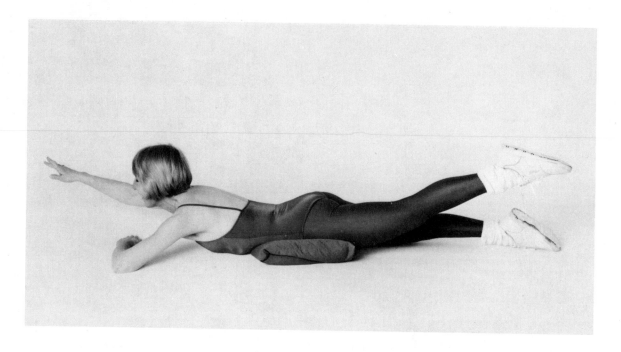

POSITION: Lie prone, with a pillow under your hips and your forehead resting on your hands.

ACTIVITY: Inhale, and then exhale as you raise your right arm and your left leg simultaneously as far up as possible. Lower down to the floor.

REPETITIONS: Repeat with other arm and leg, alternating ten times.

12. Chin and Chest Raise

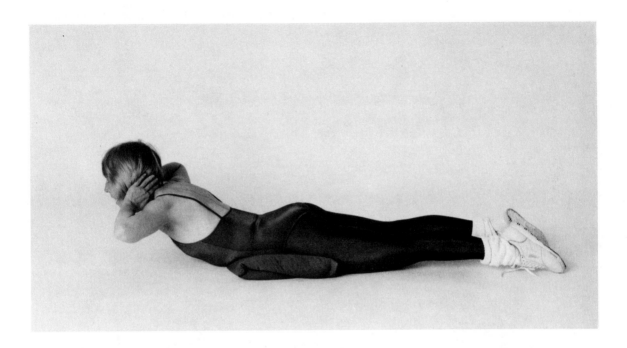

POSITION: Lie prone, with a pillow under your hips. Clasp your hands behind your head.

ACTIVITY: Inhale, and then exhale as you raise your chin and chest as far off the floor as possible. Relax down to the starting position.

REPETITIONS: Ten. Add a one-pound weight held between the hands and increase the weight gradually up to five pounds.

13. Fold up into Hip Stretch

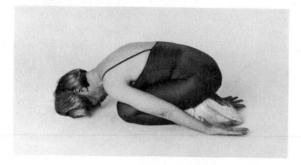

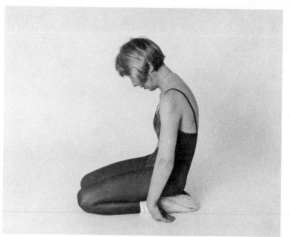

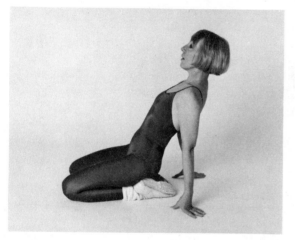

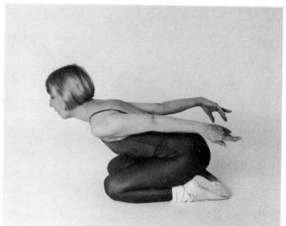

POSITION:

On your knees, with your forehead on the floor, fold up into a fetal position with your arms down along your sides.

ACTIVITY:

Roll your spine up to sitting with your buttocks resting on your heels. Place your hands on the floor behind you; inhale, and then exhale as you raise your hips up to the ceiling. Stay in this position for thirty to sixty seconds; then return to the sitting position. Bend forward and return to the fetal position.

IMAGE:

See your pelvis as the initiator of the movement as you move it to shift back onto your heels. Do not arch your back. Keep your thoughts on the front of the hip joint. Imagine that your hip joint is going to open up into a great big yawn.

REPETITIONS:

Four.

14. *Psoas Racer's Stretch*

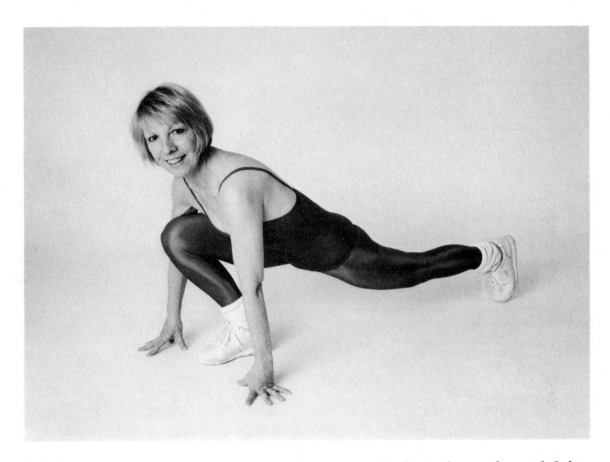

POSITION:	Lunge forward on your right leg and extend your left leg behind you. Keep directing the energy of the left hip forward to the floor. Do not allow the left buttock to protrude to the back.
ACTIVITY:	Stretch your left hip down toward the floor.
IMAGE:	See your left hip stretching and lengthening like a rubber band.
DURATION:	Thirty to sixty seconds.
	Repeat with the other leg.

15. *Knee Stretch, Hamstring Stretch, and Back Strengthener*

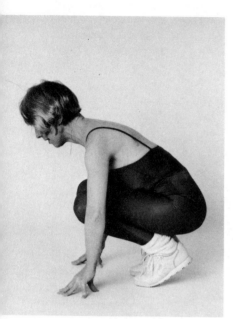 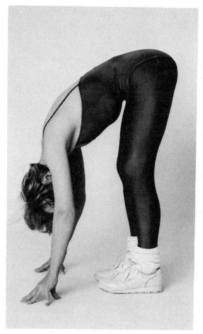 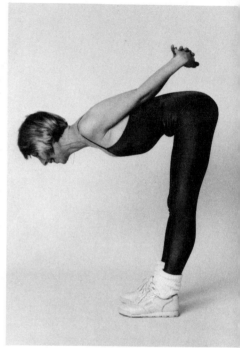

POSITION:	Squat down with both hands on the floor.
ACTIVITY 1:	Inhale, and then exhale as you stretch your buttocks up to the ceiling while keeping your hands on the floor. Keep your knees slightly bent.
ACTIVITY 2:	Clasp your hands behind your back and arch your upper back. Release and drop your hands back down to the floor and repeat.
IMAGE:	When you arch your upper back, keep your thoughts in the front of your torso, and imagine it expanding and widening out to your sides.
DURATION:	Hold each position for thirty seconds.
REPETITIONS:	Four to five times.

16. *Painter's Stretch into Hamstring Stretch*

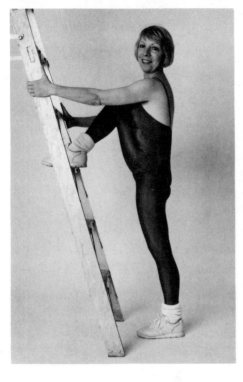
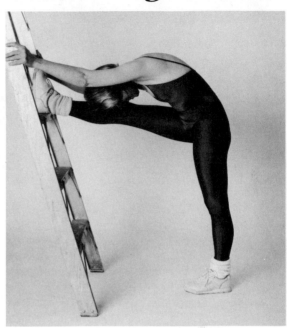

POSITION:	Stand on your left leg. Bend your right knee and place your right foot on a desk, tabletop, or ladder at a comfortable height.
ACTIVITY 1:	Push your left hip forward toward the desk.
IMAGE:	See a beam of light being projected forward from your left hip joint.
DURATION:	Thirty seconds.
ACTIVITY 2:	Hamstring stretch: Stretch your right leg forward on top of the desk. Inhale, and then exhale as you drop your head toward your right knee.
IMAGE:	As you breathe, feel the weight of the head, neck, and shoulders pull the spine forward and down to your knee, like the bough of a tree being weighted down with heavy snow.
DURATION:	Thirty seconds.
	Repeat with the other leg.

17. *Psoas Bow Stretch*

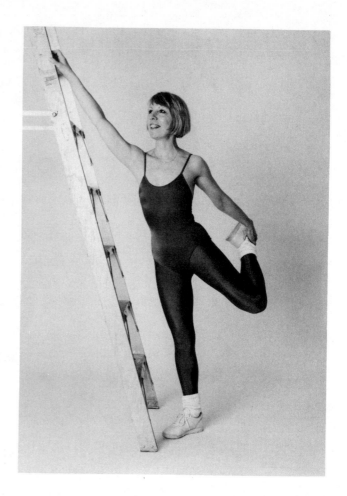

POSITION:

Stand on your right leg with your left knee bent behind you. Hold onto your left foot with your left hand. If necessary, balance yourself with your right hand against a wall, on a tabletop, and so on.

ACTIVITY:

Stretch your left leg behind you and pull it with your hand. Feel the stretch along the front of your thigh. Reach forward with your right arm for an oppositional pull.

IMAGE:

Keep your thoughts in the front of your left thigh while using the image of a bow arcing from your torso and all the way through your left thigh.

DURATION:

Thirty to sixty seconds.

Repeat with the other leg.

PERSONAL PROGRESS CHART

Basic Back Workout—Level III **EXERCISE #**

# Reps/Flexibility Level	Week #1	Week #2	Week #3	Week #4	Week #5	Week #6	Week #11	Week #12
1.								
2.								
3.								
4.								
5.								
6.								
7.								
8.								
9.								
10.								
11.								
12.								
13.								
14.								
15.								
16.								

Comments:

Workout Sequence #4

1. *Double-Knee Hug with Knee Kiss*
2. *Double-Knee Spiral Stretch with Top Leg Stretched*
3. *Single-Knee Spiral with Leg Stretch and Standing Leg Long*
4. *Hammock*
5. *Drop, Swing, Flex with Hamstring Stretch and Standing Leg Long*
6. *Psoas Release with Head Lift and Leg Stretched Long*
7. *Psoas Strengthener #2*
8. *Abdominals*
   A. *Pelvic Tilt*
   B. *Crunch with Hands Clasped Behind Head While Holding Weight*
   C. *Diagonal Crunch with Hands Clasped Behind Head While Holding Weight*
   D. *Toe Touch, Halfway Down and Legs off Floor with Head up Alternating Elbow to Knee*
   E. *Crunch with Legs up*
   F. *Pop-Up*
   G. *Pop 'n' Crunch*
9. *Knee Drop*
10. *Sitting Psoas Stretch*
11. *Psoas Stretch from All Fours to Floor and up to Wrists*
12. *Single Arm and Leg Raise/Double Arm and Leg Raise*
13. *Psoas Twist*
14. *Fold up into Hip Stretch*
15. *The Prow*
16. *Knee Stretch, Hamstring Stretch, and Back Strengthener*
17. *Painter's Stretch into Hamstring Stretch*
18. *Psoas Bow Stretch*

1. Double-Knee Hug with Knee Kiss

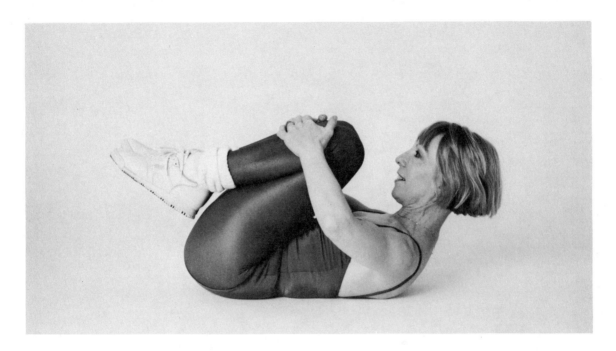

POSITION:	Lie supine, with your knees bent and your feet flat on the floor.
ACTIVITY:	Tilt your pelvis, and bring both knees toward your chest. Exhale as you gently pull your knees as close to your chest as you can. Inhale, and then exhale as you raise your head and shoulders off the floor. Bring your head and knees as close together as possible.
IMAGE:	Imagine that you are creating space and distance between each vertebra as you stretch forward to kiss your knees.
DURATION:	Thirty seconds.

2. Double-Knee Spiral with Top Leg Stretched

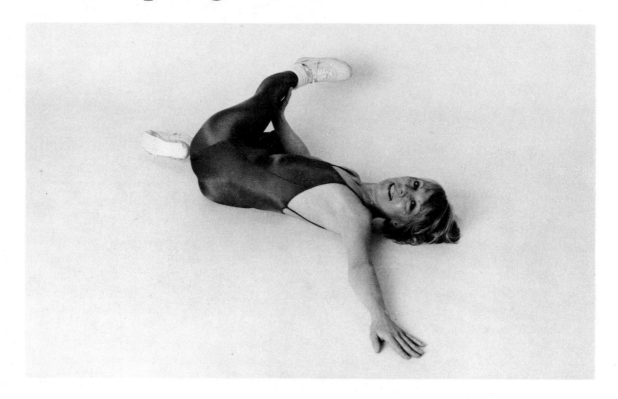

POSITION:	Lie supine, with your knees bent and your feet flat on the floor and your arms outstretched from your shoulders.
ACTIVITY:	Inhale, and then exhale as you raise both knees to your chest. Inhale, and then exhale as you lower both knees to your right side, resting them on the floor. Twist your head to the left side. Inhale, and then exhale as you stretch your top (left) leg to your right hand. Inhale, and then exhale as you bend your left knee and return to your back. Repeat on the other side.
IMAGE:	See the energy spiral through your spine and out through your leg.
DURATION:	Thirty seconds.

3. Single-Knee Spiral with Leg Stretch and Standing Leg Long

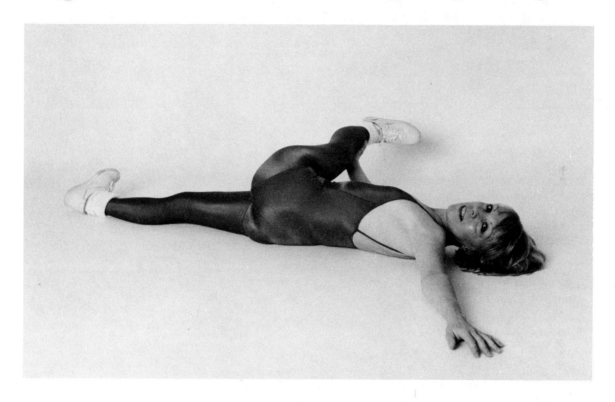

POSITION:

Lie supine, with your left knee bent to your chest, and your right leg stretched long on the floor, and your arms outstretched from your shoulders.

ACTIVITY:

Inhale and exhale as you drop your left knee over to the right side on the floor. Turn your head to the left. Inhale, and then exhale as you stretch your left leg up to your right hand.

IMAGE:

Feel the oppositional energies that are flowing through each leg. Feel the energy of the left leg go up and out into space through your left foot and the energy of your right leg flowing down and out through the right foot.

DURATION:

Thirty to sixty seconds.

Repeat with the other leg.

4. Hammock

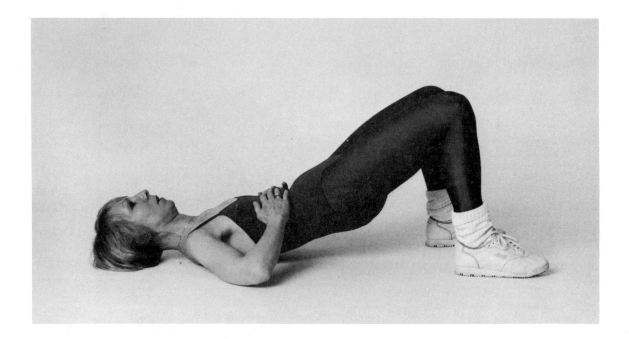

POSITION:	Lie supine, with your knees bent, and feet flat on the floor.
ACTIVITY:	Inhale, and then exhale as you slowly raise your hips up toward the ceiling. Inhale, and then exhale while slowly lowering your hips back down to the floor.
IMAGE:	Imagine that the inhalation begins at your pelvis and travels up your back. See your back opening and widening out to the sides. The exhale passes your lips, your chin, your sternum, and your rib cage and drops down into your abdominals as you raise your hips upward. Use the same image for breathing as you lower the hips to the floor.
REPETITIONS:	Four.

5. Drop, Swing, Flex with Hamstring Stretch and Standing Leg Long

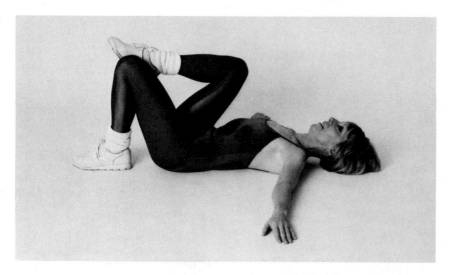

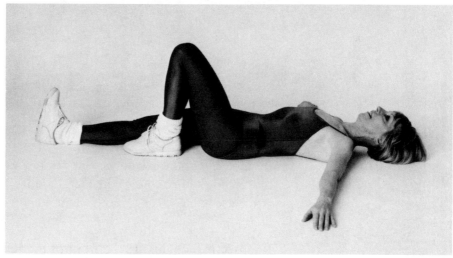

POSITION:	Lie supine, with your knees bent and your feet flat on the floor.
ACTIVITY:	Repeat drop, swing, flex as done previously on page 118. Finish with your right knee bent up to your chest. Then place both hands on your right thigh and stretch your left leg long.

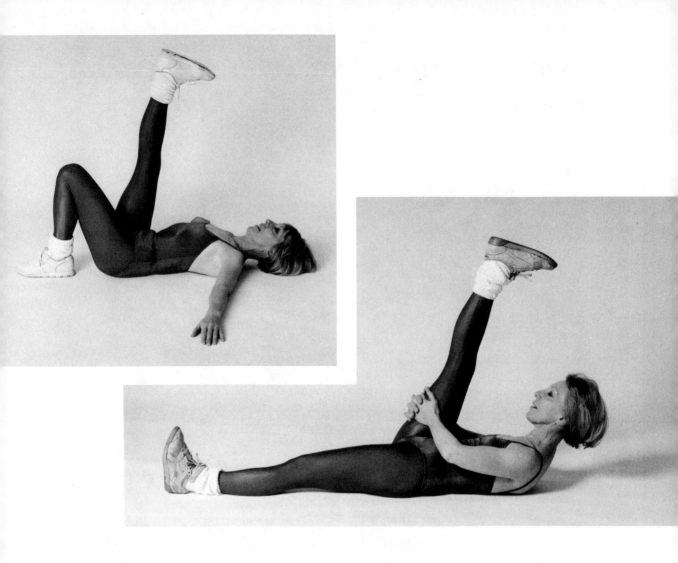

Inhale, and then exhale as you stretch your right leg up to the ceiling. Flex your right foot, inhale, and then exhale as you raise your head to your right knee. Relax down to the floor.

IMAGE:

Keep your thoughts on the front of the left thigh. When you stretch your right leg up, don't let the left thigh pop up or let the knee bend. Keep your thoughts lengthening your left leg down, energy coming from your left hip joint, through the center of your left leg, and out your left foot.

DURATION:

Thirty to sixty seconds.

Repeat with the other leg.

6. *Psoas Release with Head Lift and Leg Stretched Long*

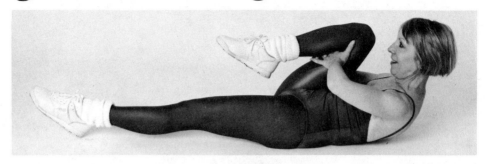

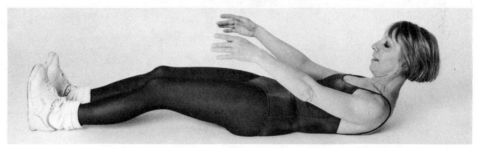

POSITION:	Lie supine, with your right knee bent to your chest and your left leg stretched long.
ACTIVITY 1:	Keep your right knee pulled up toward your chest. Inhale, and then exhale as you raise your head up to your knee. Relax down to the floor.
ACTIVITY 2:	Stretch your right leg down alongside the left leg, with both legs parallel to each other. Inhale, and then exhale as you raise your head and shoulders up. Reaching forward with your hands, bend your knees slightly so that you can press your lower back into the floor.
IMAGE:	Feel the energies of your upper and lower torso flowing to your center (abdominals and lower back) and melting down into the floor as you raise your head and reach toward your pelvis with your arms.
DURATION:	Thirty seconds.
	Repeat with the other leg.

7. Psoas Strengthener #2

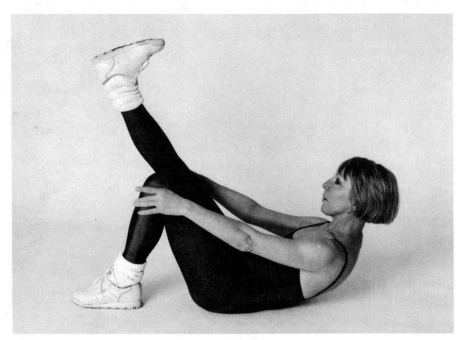

Single Straight-Leg Raises:

POSITION: Lie supine, with your knees bent and your feet flat on the floor.

ACTIVITY: Tilt your pelvis, and keep your left leg bent at both the hip and the knee. Slowly stretch the right leg and raise it to the same level as the bent knee so that both thighs are parallel. Flex the right foot and keep the leg there and inhale. Exhale and raise your head.

IMAGE: Imagine that your belly button is the central vortex through which energy swirls downward to the floor as the extended leg arcs upward to the opposite leg.

REPETITIONS: Ten.

Repeat with the other leg.

NOTE: As your strength improves, you can try adding ankle weights to the extended leg. Start with one-pound weights and gradually work up to five-pound weights.

8. *Abdominals*

A. PELVIC TILT

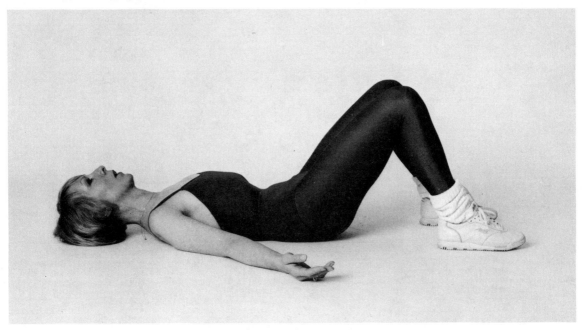

POSITION: Lie supine, with your knees bent and feet flat on the floor. Clasp your hands behind your head while holding a soft leg weight.

ACTIVITY: Inhale, and then exhale as you pull your abdomen in toward your spine while flattening the back against the floor.

IMAGE: Imagine that your belly button is a vortex, where a swirling mass of water drains down to the floor.

REPETITIONS: Ten.

B. CRUNCH WITH HANDS CLASPED BEHIND HEAD WHILE HOLDING WEIGHT

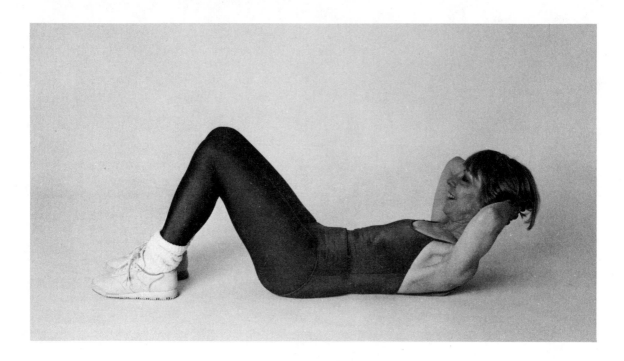

POSITION: Lie supine, with your knees bent and your feet flat on the floor. Clasp your hands behind your head while holding a soft leg weight.

ACTIVITY: Inhale, and then exhale as you tilt your pelvis and press your abdominals to the floor. Raise your head and shoulders off the floor; keep your belly button pressed to the floor. Relax down and repeat.

REPETITIONS: Ten to twenty.

NOTE: Start with a one-pound and progress up to a five-pound weight.

C. DIAGONAL CRUNCH WITH HANDS CLASPED BEHIND HEAD WHILE HOLDING WEIGHT

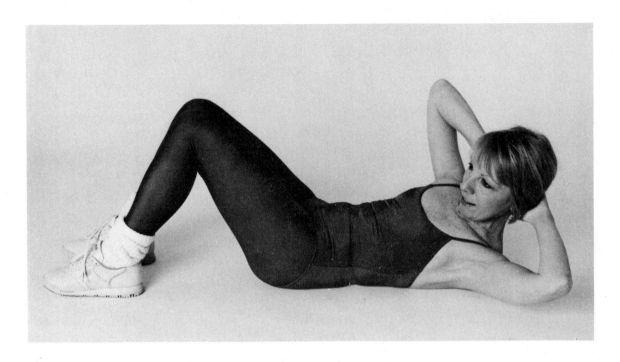

POSITION:	Lie supine, with your knees bent and your feet flat on the floor. Clasp your hands behind your head while holding a soft leg weight.
ACTIVITY:	Inhale, and then exhale as you tilt your pelvis to the floor and press your abdominals downward. Raise your head and reach your right shoulder toward your left knee. Keep your belly button pressed to the floor. Relax down and repeat.
REPETITIONS:	Ten with a right twist; ten with a left twist.
NOTE:	Start with a one-pound weight and progress up to a five-pound weight.

D. TOE TOUCH, HALFWAY DOWN AND LEGS OFF FLOOR WITH HEAD UP ALTERNATING ELBOW TO KNEE

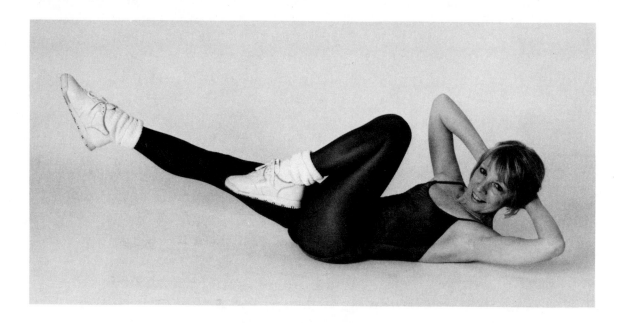

POSITION:

Lie supine, with your knees bent and raised up to your chest.

ACTIVITY:

Repeat the activities for toe touch, halfway down and legs off the floor with head up. Repeat the activity of extending your legs downward and off the floor with your head up and your hands clasped behind your head. Now bring your right elbow to your left knee. Alternate and bring your left elbow to your right knee.

REPETITIONS:

Ten to twenty.

E. CRUNCH WITH LEGS UP

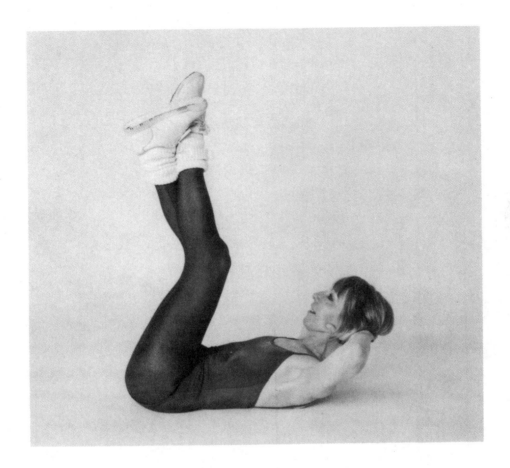

POSITION: Lie supine, with your legs partially extended to the ceiling and your feet crossed at your ankles. Clasp your hands behind your head.

ACTIVITY: Inhale, and then exhale as you raise your head, neck, and shoulders off the floor toward your legs. Keep your belly button pressed down to the floor. Relax down and repeat.

REPETITIONS: Ten to twenty.

F. POP-UP

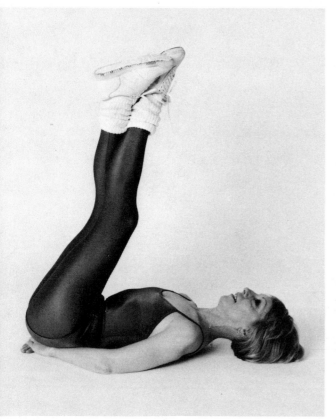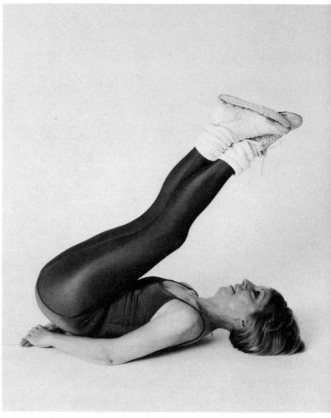

POSITION:	Lie supine, with your legs partially extended to the ceiling and your feet crossed at the ankles. Place your hands under your pelvis.
ACTIVITY:	Inhale, and then exhale as you roll your legs toward your upper torso. Feel your lower back lengthen and stretch as you gently rock your pelvis down to the floor.
REPETITIONS:	Ten to twenty.

G. POP 'N' CRUNCH

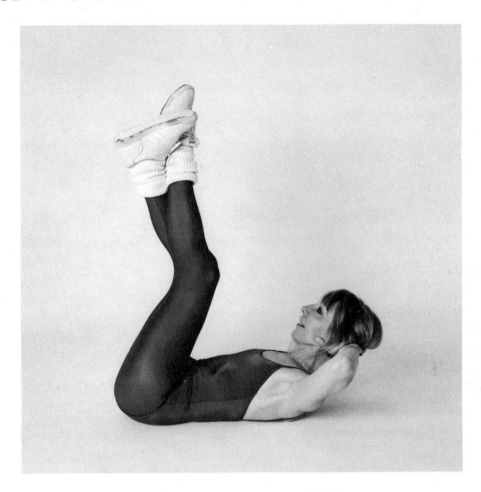

POSITION: Lie supine, with your legs partially extended to the ceiling, feet crossed at the ankles, and your hands clasped behind your head.

ACTIVITY: Roll your legs toward your upper torso as you press your tummy down to the floor. Simultaneously raise your head, neck, and shoulders off the floor toward your lower body. Remember to exhale as you crunch up.

REPETITIONS: Ten to twenty.

9. *Knee Drop*

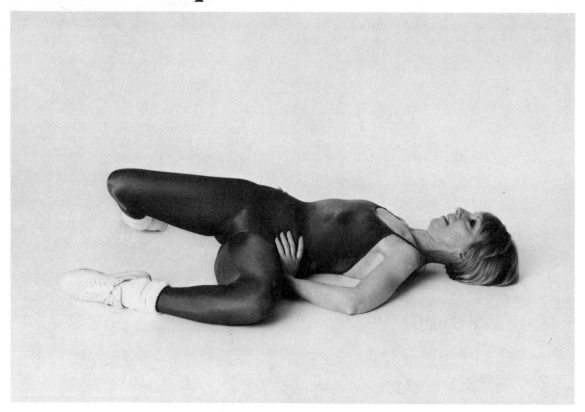

POSITION: Lie supine, with your knees bent and feet flat on the floor.

ACTIVITY: Inhale, and then exhale while dropping both knees to the floor on the left side. The left leg will turn out, and the right leg will turn in.

IMAGE: See a rotating wheel on your right pelvic crest bone. It is rotating counterclockwise toward the floor. See an opposite line of energy going from the crest bone down along the thighbone toward the knee. (This image should help to keep you from arching your lower back.)

DURATION: Thirty seconds.

              Repeat on the other side.

10. *Sitting Psoas Stretch*

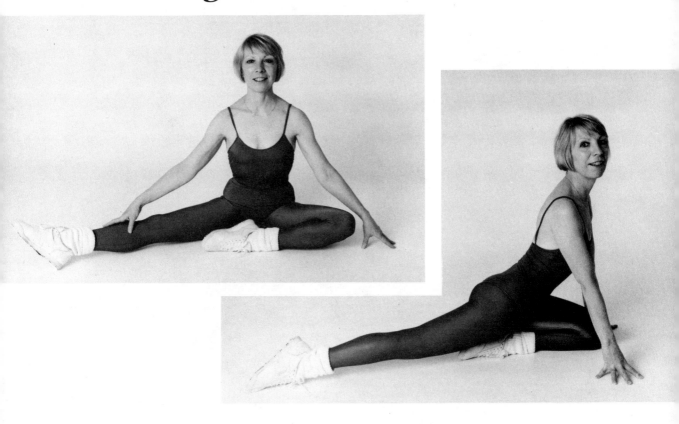

POSITION:	Sit with your legs open in a V-position.
ACTIVITY:	Bend your left knee in front of you, and shift your weight onto your left hip. Place each hand on either side of your left knee. Lift your left hip off the floor, and shift some of your weight onto your hands. Turn your right leg inward as you turn to face your left knee, and stretch your right leg behind you.
IMAGE:	Keep your thoughts concentrated on the front of your right hip (to prevent compression in the lower back). Imagine a line of energy arcing down the front of your right leg and an opposite line of energy in the front of your right hip arcing up through your vertical torso.
DURATION:	Thirty to sixty seconds.
	Repeat with your left leg.

11. *Psoas Stretch from All Fours to Floor and up to Wrists*

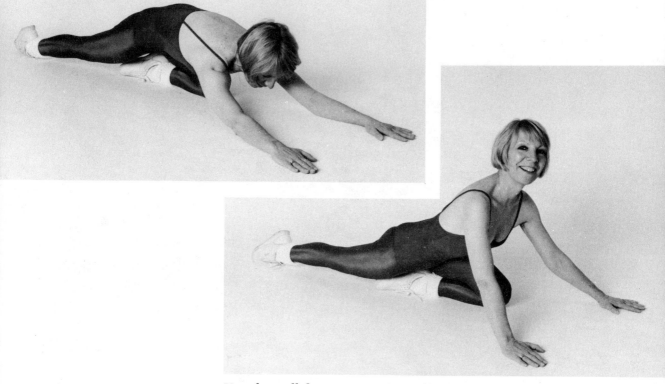

POSITION: Kneel on all fours.

ACTIVITY: Slide your right leg behind you until your head reaches the floor and your arms are stretched forward. Bend at the elbows and slide your hands back toward your left knee, placing your wrists directly under your shoulders. Straighten your elbows and push up onto your arms, shifting your torso to vertical with your weight above the right hip.

IMAGE: Imagine that you have a window in the front of your right hip. Start at the center of the window, and see yourself pushing the lower portion of the window downward and pulling the upper portion up toward the ceiling.

DURATION: Thirty to sixty seconds.

Repeat with the left leg.

12. *Single Arm and Leg Raise/ Double Arm and Leg Raise*

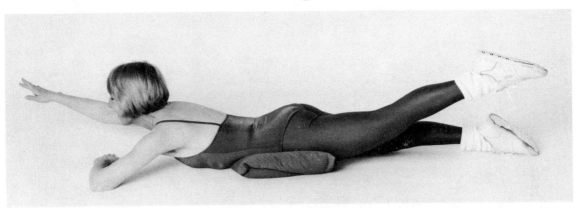

POSITION:	Lie prone, with a pillow under your hips, and extend your arms forward in a V-position on the floor.
ACTIVITY:	Inhale, and then exhale as you raise your right arm and your left leg simultaneously as far up as possible. Lower down to the floor.
REPETITIONS:	Repeat with the other arm and leg, alternating ten times.

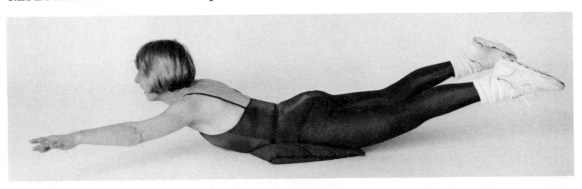

POSITION:	Lie prone, with a pillow under your hips. Extend your arms forward along the floor in a wide V-position, and spread your legs in a small V-position.
ACTIVITY:	Inhale, and then exhale as you raise both arms and both legs simultaneously as far up as possible. Lower down to the floor.
REPETITIONS:	Ten.

13. *Psoas Twist*

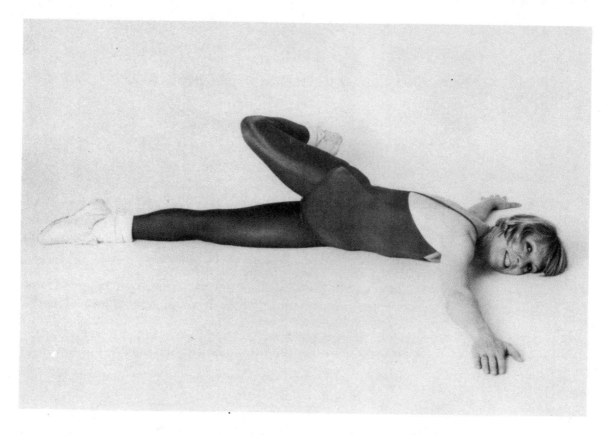

POSITION: Lie prone, with your legs together and your arms outstretched to the sides on the floor.

ACTIVITY: Lift your right leg, and bend your knee. Bring your right foot toward your left hand. Keep your shoulders on the floor.

IMAGE: Think of your right hip as being pulled forward to the floor by gravity as your right leg spirals back in the opposite direction away from the floor.

DURATION: Thirty seconds.

Repeat with the left leg.

14. *Fold up into Hip Stretch*

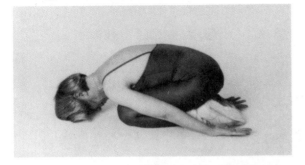

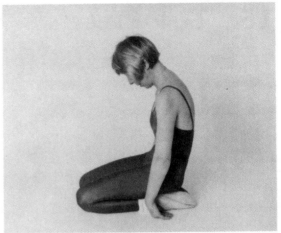

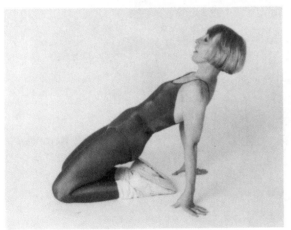

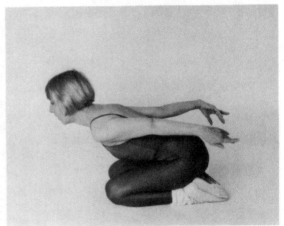

POSITION:

On your knees with your forehead on the floor, fold up into a fetal position with your arms down along your sides.

ACTIVITY:

Roll your spine up to sitting with your buttocks resting on your heels. Place your hands on the floor behind you; inhale, and then exhale as you raise your hips up to the ceiling. Stay in this position for thirty to sixty seconds, then return to the sitting position. Bend forward and return to the fetal position.

IMAGE:

See your pelvis as the initiator of the movement as you move it to shift back onto your heels. Do not arch your back. Keep your thoughts on the front of the hip joint. Imagine that your hip joint is going to open up into a great big yawn.

REPETITIONS:

Four.

15. The Prow

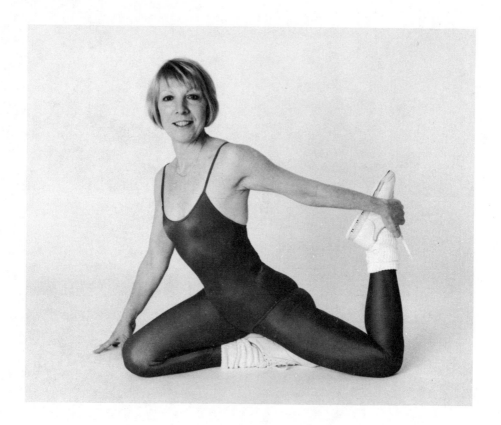

POSITION: Kneel on both knees. Slide your left leg back as you shift your weight onto your right heel.

ACTIVITY: Bend your left knee while raising your left foot to the ceiling. Hold onto your left foot with your left hand. Gently push your left hip forward toward the floor as you pull your left foot closer to your body.

IMAGE: Keep your thoughts in the front of your torso to prevent compression in the lower back. In your mind's eye, see your torso arcing forward as though you were a ship's prow.

DURATION: Thirty to sixty seconds.

Repeat with the right leg.

16. *Knee Stretch, Hamstring Stretch, and Back Strengthener*

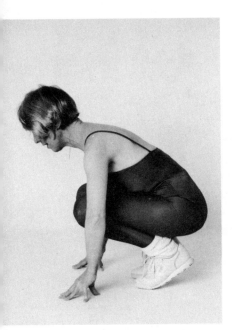
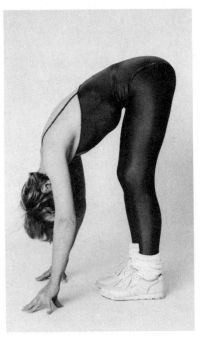
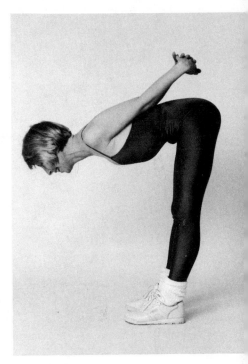

POSITION:	Squat with both hands on the floor.
ACTIVITY 1:	Inhale, and then exhale as you stretch your buttocks up to the ceiling while keeping your hands on the floor. Keep your knees slightly bent.
ACTIVITY 2:	Clasp your hands behind your back and arch your upper back. Release and drop your hands back down to the floor and repeat.
IMAGE:	When you arch your upper back, keep your thoughts in the front of your torso, and imagine it expanding and widening out to your sides.
DURATION:	Hold each position for thirty seconds.
REPETITIONS:	Four to five times.

17. Painter's Stretch into Hamstring Stretch

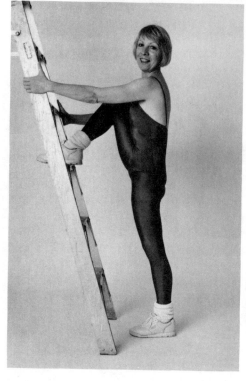
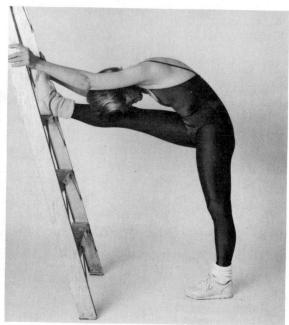

POSITION: Stand on your left leg and bend your right knee. Place your right foot on a desk, tabletop, or ladder at a comfortable height.

ACTIVITY 1: Push your left hip forward toward the desk.

IMAGE: See a beam of light being projected forward from your left hip joint.

DURATION: Thirty seconds.

ACTIVITY 2: *Hamstring stretch:* Stretch your right leg forward on top of the desk. Inhale, and then exhale as you drop your head down toward your right knee.

IMAGE: As you breathe, feel the weight of the head, neck, and shoulders pull the spine forward and down to your knee, like the bough of a tree being weighted down with heavy snow.

DURATION: Thirty seconds.

Repeat with the other leg.

18. *Psoas Bow Stretch*

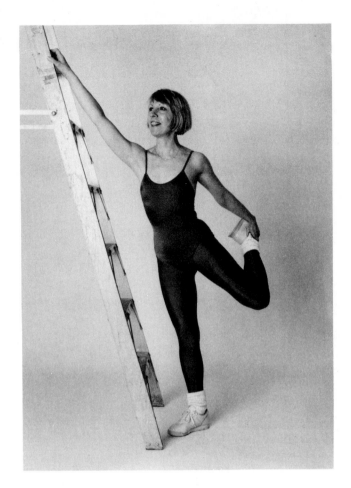

POSITION:

Stand on your right leg with your left knee bent behind you. Hold onto your left foot with your left hand. If necessary, balance yourself with your right hand against a wall, on a tabletop, and so on.

ACTIVITY:

Stretch your left leg behind you, and pull it with your hand. Feel the stretch along the front of your thigh. Reach forward with your right arm for an oppositional pull.

IMAGE:

Keep your thoughts in the front of your left thigh while using the image of a bow arcing from your torso and all the way through your left thigh.

DURATION:

Thirty to sixty seconds.

Repeat with the other leg.

PERSONAL PROGRESS CHART

Basic Back Workout—Level IV   **EXERCISE #**

# Reps/Flexibility Level	Week #1	Week #2	Week #3	Week #4	Week #5	Week #6	Week #11	Week #12
1.								
2.								
3.								
4.								
5.								
6.								
7.								
8.								
9.								
10.								
11.								
12.								
13.								
14.								
15.								
16.								

Comments:

Two-Minute Stretch
for a Stubborn Psoas

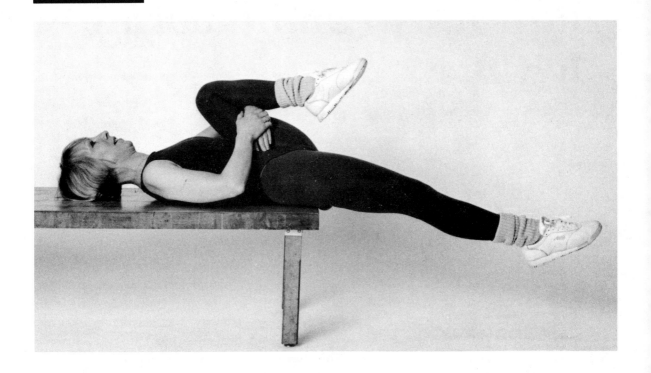

POSITION:
Lie supine on top of a desk or a table with your hips at the edge so that your legs extend beyond the surface.

ACTIVITY:
Preparation: Bend your left knee to your chest to stabilize your hip and wrap your arms around your left thigh for support. Extend your right leg to the ceiling, and then begin to let it drop down to the floor. (Make sure that your lower back does not arch up off the table.)

IMAGE:
Breathe deeply into your right hip, and imagine space and air filling the front of your right hip. Imagine a wheel rotating counterclockwise toward the table. Imagine the air at your right hip joint beginning to flow downward toward your foot.

DURATION:
Thirty to sixty seconds.

Repeat with the other leg.

5

Burn It! Fat and Calories, Bye, Bye!

THE OVERWEIGHT PERSON WITH BACK PAIN

Obesity, a condition in which a person is 20 percent or more above his or her ideal weight, is inconvenient, unhealthy, and psychologically destructive. Obesity is associated with an increased risk of high blood pressure, heart disease, stroke, hardening of the arteries, and diabetes. Being overweight not only affects your looks, it threatens your health and your feelings of self-worth. There are many serious consequences of being overweight, but since this book is about posture, proper back care, and the importance of strong abdominal muscles and an optimally functioning psoas muscle, I will contain my comments about obesity within this context.

A soft, flabby belly is a good indication that too much fat surrounds the vital organs. When a person becomes overweight, fat accumulates in the body's natural fat-storage area, located in the abdominal region. Nature provides us with a saclike area to be used in much the same way that a bear stores fat for hibernation. But since we don't hibernate, this surplus of fat won't go away unless we do something about it, such as exercise and diet control.

This excess weight in the abdominal area pulls the belly forward and can cause the pelvis to tip forward, shortening the psoas and causing strain in the lower back. Therefore, any exercise program for the overweight person with lower back problems should include an aerobic workout to burn the stored fat. The workouts in Chapter 4 should help your bad back, but the real key to total fitness is to combine them with a sensible program of aerobic exercise and diet.

Overweight people generally are not as mobile as their more fit peers, and when they exercise, their excess poundage can put extreme stress on their joints. To protect the joints, increase mobility and fitness, and burn fat, I recommend a low-impact form of aerobic activity.

AEROBIC VS. ANAEROBIC EXERCISE

Active exercise can be categorized in two groups: aerobic and anaerobic. Aerobic refers to the state that is created in the pulmonary (heart and lungs) and circulatory systems by exercise that demands oxygen to burn food or stored fat for energy.

- Activity requires energy.
- The body produces energy by burning or metabolizing food.
- The burning agent is oxygen.

FUEL = FOOD/FAT   FLAME = OXYGEN

Aerobic = with oxygen

Exercises that demand oxygen without producing oxygen debt, so that they can be sustained for long periods, are considered to be aerobic. Aerobic exercise should be at a specific level of intensity that can be monitored using your heart rate or pulse as your guide. Aerobic exercise produces several significant changes in your body: Your lungs will process more air with less effort. Your heart will pump more blood with fewer strokes. The blood supply to your muscles will improve and their volume will increase. And, last but not least, your stored fat will be burned as fuel for energy.

Our muscular system has two types of muscle fibers: red-twitch muscle fibers and white-twitch muscle fibers. Just as a turkey has dark meat and white meat, we have "dark meat" red muscle fibers and "white meat" white muscle fibers. The red muscle fibers are dark because they require a high content of iron to function. It is the red-twitch muscle fibers that burn fat, and this fat is used as a source of energy. Most fat is burned in the muscle during aerobic activity. Fat is burned from many areas: the abdomen, arms, legs, arteries, around the heart, and so on. Since the body is burning fat, carbohydrates (the other source of energy) including blood sugar are not needed to any great extent. This means that, if done properly, aerobic activity should not leave you hungry or fatigued.

Anaerobic = without oxygen

Anaerobic exercise works in another way. The white-twitch muscle fibers ("white meat") are without iron, and they require carbohydrates for energy, which lowers your blood sugar. During anaerobic exercise, fat burning stops. Hunger and fatigue often follow the exercise. An anaerobic exercise is a fast and high-stress activity (e.g., sprinting) that cannot be sustained for as long as an aerobic activity.

Two Popular Myths

1. "I get my aerobic exercise by walking to work every day." Walking is an excellent exercise, but unless you are walking at your target rate (between 120 and 170 beats per minute) steadily and consistently (without standing and waiting for the traffic light, for example) for a period of twenty to thirty minutes, you are not working aerobically. If you do walk to work, you must do it at a fast enough clip, monitor your pulse rate, and stay at it for twenty to thirty minutes.
2. "Your aerobics class isn't 'hard' enough . . . I'm accustomed to doing one hundred jumping jacks, really huffing and puffing and working up a sweat until I'm exhausted." The perception that sweating and jumping around until you are ready to drop is a really "good and hard workout" is incorrect—that is, if you want to exercise properly for aerobic conditioning. "Huffing and puffing" creates oxygen debt, which puts you over into the threshold of anaerobic metabolism, and so you receive none of the benefits of aerobic exercise.

LOW-IMPACT AEROBICS

The wear and tear that the body receives while performing high-impact exercises is very destructive. With running, for example, the impact of the feet pounding into the ground sends shock waves up through the feet, calves, thighs, hips, and back. Any vulnerable spots in your musculoskeletal system will be subjected to considerable stress, causing an array of disabling complaints such as shin splints, bone fractures, or inflamed muscles. This is made even worse if you don't have proper shoes or are running on cement.

Excessive impact is a major problem in running for fitness. There can also be unnecessary high-impacting stress with aerobic dancing as well. Some of the factors that can be stressful are nonresilient floors (cement covered with carpeting), incorrect footwear, and endless repetitions of the same activity, such as one hundred jumping jacks.

Working at too high an intensity level will not only set you up for injury but will "burn you out." You will burn out because your body will be using glucose (blood sugar, indicating anaerobic metabolism for energy). After exercising and depleting your sugar stores, you will feel wiped out rather than rejuvenated. As the intensity of the exercise increases, the proportion of body fat that is burned off actually goes *down*! When exercising aerobically, you must remain at your target rate steadily and consistently for twenty to thirty minutes in order to utilize the oxygen taken in during exercise efficiently. When exercising at heart rates between 120 and 170 beats per minute (BPM), you will be using aerobic metabolism. That means that oxygen will burn your stored fat for energy. Exercise at too high an intensity will not achieve the desired effects of training your heart, lungs, and circulatory system and burning your fat for weight loss, and it will set you up for injury in the process.

Low Impact/Low Intensity When you work at lower intensity you will enjoy yourself more. You will be able to exercise for a longer period of time. I recommend that you exercise aerobically for thirty minutes at 60 to 65 percent of your maximum heart rate rather than at 70 percent for twenty minutes.

Resting Heart Rate

To find your most accurate resting heart rate (RHR), take your pulse *before* you get out of bed in the morning. Time yourself for fifteen seconds. The average range for women is between seventy and ninety beats per minute (BPM) and for men between sixty and eighty BPM.

How to Find Your Target Heart Rate

The key to cardiovascular conditioning is to keep your heart rate in the training zone for the entire duration of the exercise (twenty to thirty minutes.) Your training zone can be determined by taking the assumed maximum heart rate (220 BPM) minus your age, which will then result in your maximum heart rate. Subtract your resting heart rate from your maximum heart rate. Then multiply this figure by 60 percent and by 70 percent. Add your resting heart rate back in to these figures. This represents your training or target heart-rate range.

The example below illustrates the training or target heart rate for a thirty-five-year-old:

	60%	70%
Assumed maximum capacity	220	220
Age	− 35	− 35
Maximum heart rate =	185	185
Resting heart rate	− 70	− 70
	115	115
	× .60	× .70
	69.00	80.50
Resting heart rate	+ 70	+ 70
	139.00	150.50 BPM

Low-Impact Aerobics Means:

- Fat-burning, heart-working aerobic activity without the shocking stress to the muscles and joints.
- Continuous rhythmic action of the power muscles in your back, buttocks, and thighs.
- Movement that is low to the ground with repeated bending to work the large leg muscles.

- One foot must always remain on the floor.
- Increased armwork predominantly above the heart.
- A combination of muscle strength and aerobics, because the lower, slower movement uses muscle strength rather than momentum.
- A slower and easier pace that allows for a longer workout.
- Staying in the target range more consistently and working longer without the pulse dips and surges.
- Working aerobically at 60 to 70 percent of maximum capacity for thirty minutes, four times per week.

For more information on low-impact aerobics, see the Suggested Reading section.

ALTERNATING AEROBIC EXERCISE

Guidelines released by the American College of Obstetrics and Gynecologists (ACOG) during the Summer of 1986 indicate that impact workouts for anyone should not exceed thirty minutes and should not be done on consecutive days.

If you choose to perform low-impact aerobic exercises, alternate your workout with one of lesser intensity. Give your body a day of rest between workouts. On your off day go in for some nonimpact activity such as swimming, bicycling, or low-impact walking.

Choosing Your Alternate Aerobic Exercise

Choose an exercise that you know you will enjoy. That way you will be more likely to continue to perform that exercise on a regular basis. Alternate two or three different aerobic activities for variety and to achieve a more balanced use of the muscles in your body.

Swimming
Swimming has the advantage of the buoyancy of the water, which reduces pressure on the bones and joints of the body. The support of the body by the water takes the pressure off of the joints, which are nonweight bearing. For this reason, swimming is an excellent exercise for the obese person or the

person with musculoskeletal or lower back problems.

Another advantage of swimming is that the body's position in the water allows the blood to be returned to the heart easily. To achieve your aerobic conditioning, swim for twenty to thirty minutes, three to four times per week.

Start out with a slow, easy stroke, such as the breaststroke, and build your pulse up gradually until you reach your target heart rate. Later in the workout, you can switch to more intense strokes, such as the crawl or the butterfly.

People with weight or lower back problems will find exercising in the water very enjoyable. Even nonswimmers can benefit from aerobic exercise in a pool. You can walk back and forth in about four or five feet of water while you swing your arms back and forth. Or you can even just bounce yourself up and down in the water. Just move around and have fun!

Bicycling

Bicycling is a good form of exercise for cardiovascular conditioning if you don't have knee problems. Bicycling does an excellent job of toning the muscles of the lower body including the calves, thighs, and derriere, but it will do very little for you above the waist. If a full body workout is a must for you, try using light free weights as you ride on a stationary bike.

If you have lower back problems, you might be interested in trying the most recent state-of-the-art, semirecumbent bike. You sit on a more comfortable seat with your legs extended forward rather than downward, similar to the way you sit when driving a car, which puts considerably less strain on the lower back.

When bicycling out of doors, don't be concerned about the mileage you have covered. Instead, your goal should be to keep your heart working in your target range for twenty to thirty minutes. If you reach a hill that would increase your heart rate beyond your target range, get off your bike and walk up. Avoid long downhill rides during which your heart rate may drop below your training zone.

Aerobic Walking

Racewalking uses the muscles of the upper body as well as

the lower body. The specific form required for this activity is that one foot must be on the ground at all times. To learn more about this activity, please refer to the Suggested Reading section at the back of this book.

Walkers may choose to carry weights to increase the intensity of the exercise. When weights are combined with hill climbing and a rapid pace, an aerobic walk can expend just as much energy as running and with considerably less impact.

DIET TIPS

This is an exercise book that supports the premise that exercise is the most important element in weight control and fitness —the element that will help you attain a healthier back. It's not my purpose to write a diet book, but since poor eating habits, attitudes, and misinformation can sabotage your exercise program, let me say a few words about diet, nutrition, and food. For more information, please consult the Suggested Reading section at the back of this book.

Much of what was formerly thought about weight control, calorie counting, fad diets, and pills is now known to be nonsense. Genetics determines your body type and also, in part, how the hypothalamus in your brain will determine your particular level of fatness. This level is called your natural setpoint. Your own body and its condition will determine your weight and percentage of body fat.

The setpoint can be changed, however; eating an increased amount of rich foods, inactivity, or even dieting may increase the level at which your body maintains fat. With some diets the body may be fooled into thinking it is starving itself, and so it prepares for the famine by lowering the metabolism and maintaining a higher level of body fat in order to protect itself. Dieting is a rebellion against the body. Hormonal changes during dieting can actually lower your metabolism so that you burn calories more slowly.

Dieting alone will not change your setpoint. Daily exercise or activity, especially an aerobic workout, can lower your setpoint. But in order to maintain the lowered setpoint, you must make the exercise or activity a regular part of your daily regimen, or at least four to five times per week. Anything less than three times per week is better than nothing, although it is relatively worthless in terms of changing your metabolism.

Nutritionally Ignorant vs. Nutritionally Educated

People reveal their nutritional ignorance when they accept diet plans that promise fast weight loss with single foods or a combination of foods; diets that omit other food groups than sugar, salt, or fat; diets that claim to have special calorie-burning capabilities; or diet plans that make food and menu choices for them, which do not teach them to learn how to make their own choices. And since most physicians have had only a few hours of nutrition education, they seem to be incapable of refuting these quasi-scientific theories that purport to provide quick weight loss.

What we need is more and better nutrition education, instead of another fad diet for weight loss. We must learn that a diet is our daily food plan, not something to go on for a few months and then go off when we think we are finished. We must learn how to make permanent changes in our eating habits to keep our weight down for our whole lifetime. We must take responsibility for ourselves in making intelligent decisions regarding our eating habits. We must learn how to make the proper food selection for the best nutritional balance and the most enjoyment. We must recognize that to make lasting changes in our eating behavior, it will take at least six months or longer. Weight loss for a lifetime is a continuing and ongoing process. Your chosen food plan must be one that you can happily remain on for the rest of your life.

What You Should Not Do To Lose Weight

1. Do not take drugs, diuretics, appetite suppressants, or any other pills.
2. Do not buy specially formulated "diet" powders, liquids, or foods.
3. Do not follow a "fad" diet. (Weight loss can be quick, but it is usually temporary. Some "fad" diets can be medically dangerous.)
4. Do not fast or skip meals. (Skipping meals can lead to snacking on less nutritious foods. And, more importantly,

fasting can force the body to burn or metabolize muscle tissue for energy.)

What You Should Do To Lose Weight

1. Set weight-loss goals of one to no more than two pounds per week. Pace yourself for the long haul.
2. Reduce your caloric intake, and increase your caloric usage. A sensible plan reduces calories, does not leave out essential nutrients, and must include aerobic exercise.
3. The exercise of choice must fit in with your life-style and must be aerobic to burn fat.
4. Keep yourself active. You don't necessarily have to "exercise" to stay in shape. Some activities that require as much energy as riding a bicycle include yardwork, chopping firewood, working in the garden, or washing windows.

Diet Do's

1. *Develop your own eating plan.*
   - Be aware of the foods that are especially caloric and try to avoid or minimize them, but don't count calories.
   - Your food plan should be flexible and offer a wide range of food choices each day. Your plan should be a framework or a grid that allows you to "mix and match" food groups easily.
   - Eat whole foods, not processed foods. Our bodies did not evolve on such foods as sugary processed cereals or refined white flour; eat whole grains.
   - Eat foods rich in complex carbohydrates, such as grains, rice, cereal, beans, bread, potatoes, fruits, and vegetables. These foods allow you to eat a greater quantity with fewer calories, and they provide the fiber to keep your digestive tract working properly.
   - Eat foods as close to their natural state as possible. For example, it is healthier to eat your vegetables steamed or stir-fried rather than boiled to a pulp.
   - Eat seasonal foods. In wintertime eat hearty soups and stews, and in summertime go lighter with salads.
   - Eat local foods. Foods that are close to the source are fresher because they don't have to be shipped great distances.

- Eat foods with the correct proportion of nutrients. Refer to the Suggested Reading listings on nutrition to learn how to design meals with the proper proportion of carbohydrates, fat, and protein.

2. *Drink lots of water.*   Water purges the body of toxic waste products that accumulate as you burn body fat. Water has no calories, and since it can fill you up, it helps you to control the amount you eat.

3. *Enjoy your food plan, because you're going to use it often.*   Make sure your food plan allows you to feel good. It should be well balanced and delicious. You should not feel ravenously hungry or tired or weak. You should feel great! Better than ever!

Diet Don'ts

1. *Avoid fad diets.*   The faster you lose weight, the faster you gain it back. When you lose weight, you lose both muscle and fat. When you gain the weight back you gain fat rather than muscle.

2. *Avoid fasting.*   If you fast, your body will start digesting your muscle to get nutrients. It's like burning your house (your structure) instead of firewood (your fat) for fuel.

3. *Avoid large meals.*   Eat smaller, more frequent meals. Since the body needs only one hundred calories per hour to maintain itself, a nibbling or grazing life-style, one in which you take in small amounts of food several times a day, keeps the body from storing excess calories as fat.

4. *Avoid the following:*   sugar and concentrated sweeteners, fatty meats, cheeses, avocados, and olives; refined white flour and white rice; food additives; salt; caffeine, tobacco, and excessive alcohol.

CHANGING OUR ATTITUDES

We seem to cling to the notion that overeating, not inactivity, is the major cause of our being overweight. It seems so much easier to diet rather than to set aside a time for exercise. Most of us feel that we just don't have the time or find it difficult to make time for exercise, yet we find time to read books about weight loss and spend time perfecting low-calorie recipes. We think that since we must eat to stay alive, we might as well figure out a better way of doing it without increasing our weight gain. This is very commendable. However, we must also move and exercise to stay alive and function optimally. We would never think of not sleeping or resting. But we do think that we don't have the time to "work" our bodies. Life is a system of balances. We have night and day, inhalation and exhalation, and therefore, we must have rest and exertion. Remember the energy in (food) must equal the energy out (exercise), or it all gets stored as fat.

Spend time reevaluating your thoughts about diet and exercise. Begin to set your goals and find a practical, easy means to your end. Maybe it's true that with dieting or drastic caloric cutback, you can see the results more quickly and drop five pounds in a week. But you must realize that those five pounds will be back as soon as you start eating and drinking normally again. Changing your diet alone is *not* the key to fitness and permanent weight loss.

When following an exercise regimen, you see and feel the results much more slowly. That's why it may seem so discouraging. You don't seem to be making any progress. In fact, your weight may seem to stay the same while you are exercising and dieting, but that is because you are building muscle tissue. Muscle weighs more than fat, so that even as you are burning fat you are increasing your muscle bulk and can't see that change on your scale. Stick with your exercise program! Recent research indicates that people who both diet and exercise keep their weight off for a longer period of time. You will see the results:

- You can eat without gaining weight.
- You will feel more energized and be more productive.
- You will look better and improve your appearance.
- You will feel the release of exercise and lessen your level of emotional tension and psychological stress.
- You will increase your stamina and be able to stay with physical exertion for a longer period of time.
- You will improve your self-image, outlook on life, and overall health.

Changing Your Life-Style   In the process of changing your life-style to include more physical exertion, remember that little things add up. Here are some suggestions to get you moving:

- Walk up stairs rather than take an elevator.
- Carry your groceries rather than have them delivered.
- Walk to work rather than drive.
- Park your car at the end of the parking lot instead of in front of the store.
- Use time well while waiting in lines by performing some simple exercise such as moving your shoulders forward and back or circling your head around.
- Stretch whenever you get a chance—as you reach up to your cupboard or as you reach for items in your shopping cart.
- On the telephone a lot? Here's a great chance for you to exercise, and no one can even see you doing it. Lie down on your back and stretch your hamstrings.

There are no excuses for not getting more movement, exercise, and fun in your life. So let's get to it . . . and BURN IT! FAT AND CALORIES, BYE, BYE!

Pregnancy and the Psoas

Most pregnant women experience lower back pain, which is directly related to the part played by the psoas in the abnormal inclination of the pelvis. In his book *Iliopsoas*, orthopedic surgeon Arthur A. Michele, M. D., writes that a person who is not properly posturally aligned brings abnormal pressure upon the blood vessels at the point where they cross the psoas shelf, which can cause pain. He notes that this is particularly the case in obesity and during pregnancy. In fact, the pregnant woman is in a state of temporary pelvic imbalance until the baby is delivered.

During pregnancy the body has to adapt to hormonal changes, which affect the stability of the joints, and to structural changes, which alter its center of gravity. Accordingly, the alignment and balance of the body must also adapt to these changes. It is the position of the pelvis that supports the spine, and it is the psoas in its freely movable state that allows the proper pelvic angle. The spinal column forms an S-curve around the center line of gravity. The more exaggerated the curve, the more muscle work is necessary to keep the spine upright. During pregnancy the pelvis naturally tends to angle forward as the body's center of gravity moves forward as a result of the increased weight of the abdominal contents. If the forward tilt of the pelvis is prolonged, the muscles in the lower back will shorten and become tense and the abdominal muscles in front will stretch. With the increasing size of the abdominal contents and the stretch of the abdominal muscles, the bones and ligaments become overloaded because the muscles can no longer do their share of the workload.

To prevent this stressful compression in the lower back and the weakening in the abdomen, a pregnant woman must stretch the psoas, which begins in the lower back at the lumbar vertebrae and connects to the inside of the inner thighbone at the lower portion of the abdomen. Any instructions to "tilt the pelvis back" or "pull down the back with the buttocks muscles" will only result in further complicating the problem because of all the compensatory movements and actions that will occur.

It is the psoas that maintains the fetus in the upper abdomen, and it is the relaxation of the psoas that allows the fetus to drop into the pelvis. The squatting position for delivery releases the pull of the psoas. An attempt to simulate this posture on the obstetric table is made by bending the thighs to the pelvis.

One goal of prenatal exercise should be to develop better postural habits that will enable you to better carry the load of pregnancy. Exercises to achieve this aim will also help to stretch the psoas and strengthen the other muscles to help prevent much of the discomfort of backache that plagues most pregnant women.

It is essential for you to consult your physician as soon as you know you are pregnant. Discuss your medical and obstetric history, your current exercise regime, and the exercises you would like to continue throughout pregnancy. Any exercise prescription should be based on this medical and exercise history to minimize any complications that may occur during the pregnancy. The main determinants of appropriate exercise or training during pregnancy are a woman's pre-pregnancy fitness and her activity levels.

Most of the studies that have been done on the effect of exercise on pregnant women have used well-trained athletes as subjects. Accordingly, more guidelines are necessary for the average woman who has had little or no exercise experience. Essentially these women should be encouraged to start an exercise program prior to conception, and they should seek help from their physician in determining an exercise routine that is well within their limit of tolerance, especially if they have not been exercising regularly.

Pregnant women usually can continue their regular level of exercise during the first and second trimesters (providing it is not a high-intensity aerobic activity), but they should be aware that they will experience a gradual decrease in efficiency and performance during the second trimester. The final three months must be approached on an individual basis, and you should consult your physician about which type of exercise best suits your needs at that time. Frequent stretching exercises and short walks would be more than adequate for most women. Serious exercising can generally be started again six weeks postpartum.

Studies done on pregnant women have demonstrated that the average woman can increase her level of fitness apparently without any deleterious effects. Most of this information is based on the normal woman's response to exercise, but relatively little is known about the response of the fetus to exercise. Of particular concerns are the effects of increased body temperature and oxygen deprivation on the fetus.

There are many physiological effects of pregnancy and their implications pertaining to exercise. We will address ourselves to the following:

1. The enlarged uterus that accentuates pelvic lordosis or swayback.
2. The increased hormone levels and their effects on the joints.

EXERCISE DURING PREGNANCY—
BASIC DO'S AND DON'TS

If you have been exercising prior to your pregnancy, it will probably be all right for you to continue in the same manner but with a few modifications. If you have not been exercising before your pregnancy, it is generally not recommended that you start a vigorous program at this time. Consult your physician for specific recommendations.

For the women who have been exercising prior to pregnancy, I suggest the following: During the first two trimesters (0–24 weeks), keep your exercise as steady and consistent as you possibly can. Intermittent and sporadic exercise will not achieve the desired benefits of increased strength and flexibility. Since current research on exercising during pregnancy does not indicate the effects of increased body temperature on the fetus, high-intensity aerobic activity is not recommended. Instead, mild to moderate exercise at 50 to 60 percent of maximum capacity (90–120 heartbeats per minute) is suggested. High-intensity aerobic activities such as running, cross-country skiing, or aerobic dancing should be replaced by walking, swimming, or stationary cycling.

Since tremendous changes take place during the third trimester (24–40 weeks), the exercise program should be tailored to the individual based on how the woman feels at this time, and the complications or lack of them at this stage of the pregnancy. Of special consideration is toxemia. Toxemia can occur in the second or third trimester. The criteria for toxemia is an elevated blood pressure of the systolic at 140 or above and the diastolic at 90 or above (i.e., 140/90 as the baseline), or simply a rise of 30 points over your baseline systolic and/or 15 points over your baseline diastolic pressure. In addition to elevated blood pressure, other indications for toxemia include protein in the urine and swelling of the face, hands, and ankles. Bed rest while blood pressure is elevated will help to prevent toxemia in many, but not all, cases.

A sedentary healthy woman with no pregnancy-related problems can generally exercise twenty to forty minutes per day, every other day, or at least three times per week at an intensity of 50 to 60 percent of maximal heart rate (90–120 beats per minute).

Your exercise program should be moderate, not prolonged or exhaustive. If you need a nap afterward, you're probably doing too much. Try limiting your activity to shorter intervals. Exercise for ten or fifteen minutes, and then rest for two or three minutes. Resume exercise again for another ten or fifteen minutes. Decrease your exercise level as your pregnancy progresses. Because your greater body weight calls for a larger energy output, you will feel more fatigued.

Take your pulse every ten minutes while you are exercising. You can take your pulse by placing three fingers just to the side of your throat on your carotid artery, or you can place two fingers on the radial artery at your wrist. If your pulse is more than 140 beats per minute, slow down until it returns to the 90 to 120 range. Avoid becoming overheated for extended periods. It's best not to exercise for more than thirty-five minutes in hot, humid weather.

Avoid risky activities such as waterskiing, surfing, mountain-climbing, racquetball, and aerobic dancing. Your increasing weight along with the shift in your center of gravity and the softening of the ligaments may alter your coordination. Consider decreasing weight-bearing activities (jogging and running) and focus on nonweight-bearing activities such as swimming, stationary cycling, or stretching. Reduce your exercise sharply four weeks before your due date.

Rest for ten minutes after exercising, lying on your left side. Lying on your left side takes the pressure off the vena cava, a major vein carrying blood to your heart on your right side. It also promotes the return of circulation from your extremities and muscles to your heart, increasing blood flow to your placenta and fetus.

Drink two or three eight-ounce glasses of water after you exercise, to replace the body fluids you have lost through perspiration. While exercising, drink water whenever you feel the need.

Stop exercising *immediately* if you experience shortness of breath, dizziness, numbness, tingling, abdominal pain, or bleeding, and consult your physician at once.

THE BACK CONTROVERSY

Many exercises for the lower back and abdominal muscles involve lying on the back in the supine position. The American College of Obstetricians and Gynecologists (ACOG), however, has issued guidelines for exercise during pregnancy that specifically state: "No exercise should be performed in the supine position after the fourth month of gestation is completed." In pregnancy there is a significant change in blood pressure and heart rate. Lying supine can cause the uterus to press on the vena cava and significantly reduce the blood supply to the uterus, and thus the fetus will respond with decreased heartbeats.

However, some gynecologist-obstetricians believe that these problems are not as common as the ACOG guidelines imply and that most pregnant women can tolerate lying on their backs, at least for brief periods. These guidelines will doubtless change with time and further research, and so in the meantime the best advice is to use common sense. I would recommend the following: The exercises in the supine position can be performed through the fourth month of gestation. After that time, switch to the next series of exercises I've outlined, and don't remain on your back for any longer than twenty minutes at a stretch. Then roll onto your left side and slowly come up to sitting. If at any time you feel dizzy or out-of-sorts while on your back, stop exercising, roll onto your left side, and come up to sitting.

Exercise during pregnancy should emphasize breathing, relaxation, and stretching for proper alignment. The strengtheners should include exercises for the abdominals, the muscles of the pelvic floor, and the legs. Since it is the purpose of this book to address ourselves to the elimination of back pain (and in this chapter its eradication during pregnancy and postpartum) I will limit myself to discussing stretches for the psoas (pages 188, 200, and 212) and the lower back (pages 191, 192, 193, 203, 204, 205, 215, 216, 217) as well as abdominal strengtheners (pages 194, 196, 197, 206, 208, 209, 218, 219). Exercises for breathing and relaxation (pages 190, 202, and 214) can be used, but remember to take into consideration the ACOG guidelines to avoid the supine position after the fourth month of pregnancy.

Exercise During Pregnancy—Do's

1. Stretch your psoas and lower back to prevent lower back pain and compression. Exercises on pages 188, 200, and 212 are for the psoas. Exercises on pages 191, 192, 193, and 203, 204, 205, 215, 216, 217 are for the lower back.
2. Do exercises to strengthen your abdominal muscles. Inelastic and weak abdominals have a reduced ability to protect the joints of the pelvis and support its contents and

to help in the expulsion of the baby. Weak abdominal muscles may also predispose the rectus abdominus to separation during the strain of labor and delivery (diastasis). Exercises on pages 194, 196, 197, and 206, 208, 209, 218, 219 are for the abdominals.

3. Always perform the abdominal exercise on the exhale. When you inhale, the diaphragm lengthens downward, forcing the abdominal contents outward as the pressure increases. Therefore, if you inhale or hold your breath on the exertion, as the diaphragm moves down, your belly will bulge outwardly. Upon exertion, you always want your belly button to be pressing in toward your spine, which happens naturally on the exhalation.

4. Relaxation and proper breathing should become a habit, something you can fall back on automatically. A woman who has learned to relax by using her body during pregnancy will handle the pain of delivery with greater ease, since pain is intensified with tension. Do perform the relaxation and breathing exercise on pages 190, 202, and 214.

5. The hormonal changes that occur during pregnancy allow the ligaments to soften to permit the opening of the pelvis, and this increases your vulnerability to minor strains in the joints. Perform exercise with care and caution.

6. Since your center of gravity is shifted slightly forward you will have a tendency to lean backward. Do strive for good alignment habits, abdominal strength, and a freely functioning psoas to maintain proper posture and prevent lower back strain.

7. Be in touch with your body. It enhances your feeling about being able to surrender to the changes that are happening within your body during pregnancy. Enjoy the psychological aspects of "letting go" and flowing along with what is occurring during this time. You will accept and feel good about yourself and the way you look.

Exercise During Pregnancy—Don'ts

Prenatal exercise is not recommended in the following cases:

1. If you have not been physically active prior to pregnancy, don't start a program at this time unless your physician recommends a specific regimen.

2. If you have a history of heart disease.
3. If you are having any trouble during your pregnancy.
4. If you are going to have a multiple birth (i.e., twins).
5. If your blood pressure is elevated, especially in the third trimester, since this may indicate complications such as toxemia.
6. If you've had a history of miscarriages.
7. If you have medical conditions such as anemia, diabetes, obesity, or thyroid disease. Consult your physician before attempting physical activity during pregnancy.

Prenatal Exercise

FIRST TRIMESTER

1. *Psoas Racer's Stretch*
2. *Pelvic Floor Exercise*
3. *Deep Abdominal Breathing*
4. *Pelvic Tilt in Supine Position*
5. *Pelvic Tilt with Legs Long and Knees Soft*
6. *The Hammock*
7. *Transverse Abdominals*
8. *Forward Curl-up, Arms Reach Forward*
9. *Diagonal Curl-up, Arms Reach Forward*
10. *Repeat: Psoas Racer's Stretch*

1. *Psoas Racer's Stretch*

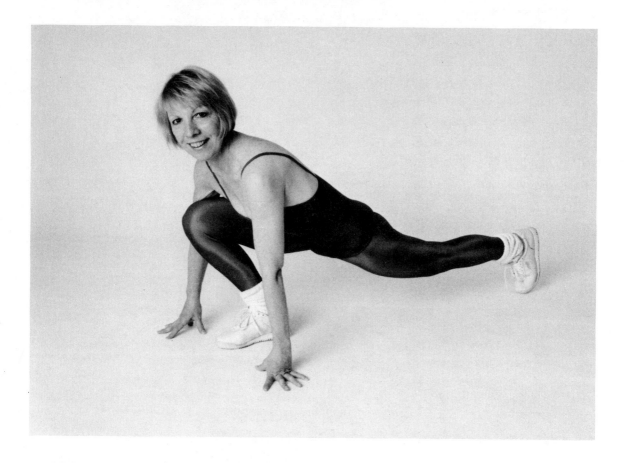

POSITION: Lunge forward on your right leg, and extend your left leg behind you. Keep your right knee over your right foot.

ACTIVITY: Stretch your left hip down toward the floor.

IMAGE: See your left hip stretching and lengthening like a rubber band.

DURATION: Thirty to sixty seconds.

Repeat with the other leg

2. *Pelvic Floor Exercise*
(DURING ENTIRE PREGNANCY AND POSTPARTUM)

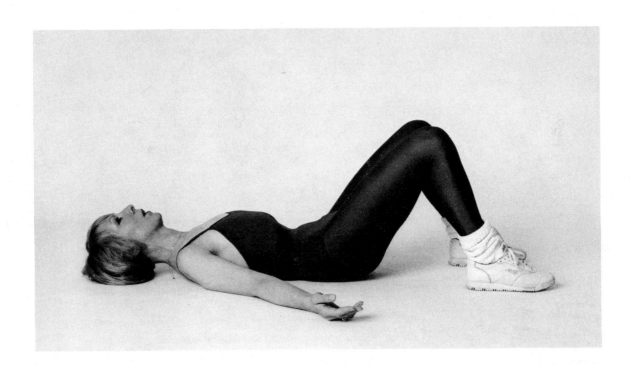

POSITION:	Lie supine, with your knees bent and your feet flat on the floor, or sit comfortably in any position.
ACTIVITY:	You should feel several muscle groups working together—your bladder, rectum, and vagina (called the perineum). (It should feel as though you are trying to stop or control urination.) Release and let go.
IMAGE:	Think of "lifting from within and pulling up to your center." Release the innermost spaces first and then the perineum.
REPETITIONS:	Twenty to fifty.
NOTE:	After you have gained proficiency, hold for a count of five and release. Repeat ten to twenty times.

3. Deep Abdominal Breathing

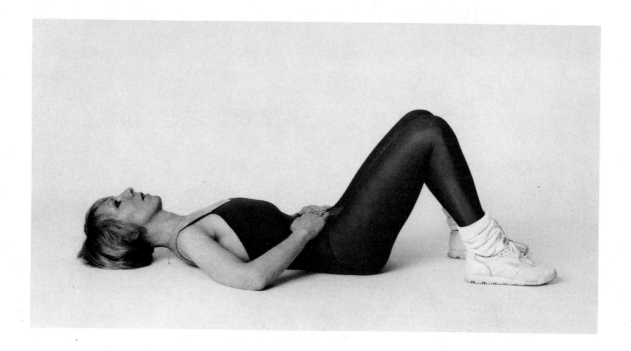

POSITION:

Lie supine, with your knees bent and your feet flat on the floor. Place your hands on your abdominal area.

ACTIVITY:

Inhaling through your nose, feel your tummy raise up to the ceiling. Continue your inhalation, slowly and deeply. Don't rush it to avoid getting dizzy. When you feel ready to exhale, allow your lips to part slightly and let the breath pass your lips, chin, collarbone, sternum, rib cage, diaphragm, and all the way down to the abdominal area. Repeat this process several times.

IMAGE:

Imagine your breath encompassing and gently caressing your baby.

DURATION:

Three to five minutes.

4. *Pelvic Tilt in Supine Position*

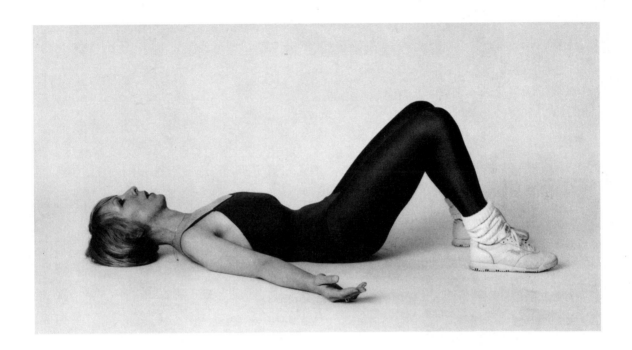

POSITION:	Lie supine, with your knees bent and your feet flat on the floor.
ACTIVITY:	Inhale, and then exhale as you pull your abdomen in toward your spine while flattening the back against the floor.
IMAGE:	Imagine that your belly button is a vortex where a swirling mass of water drains down to the floor.
REPETITIONS:	Ten.

5. *Pelvic Tilt with Legs Long and Knees Soft*

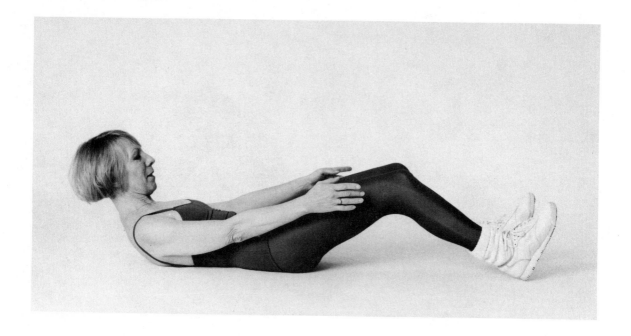

POSITION:

Lie supine, with your knees bent and your feet flat on the floor.

ACTIVITY:

1. Inhale. As you exhale, press your abdominals down to the floor as you stretch your legs long underneath you. Try to keep your lower back pressed to the floor as long as you can.

2. Inhale. As you exhale, press your abdominals down to the floor and bend your knees and ankles slightly. Raise your head, neck, and shoulders off the floor. Repeat several times.

IMAGE:

On the inhalation, see the spine and legs stretching away from each other in opposite directions just like an accordion. On the exhalation, see the energy of the spine and legs converging to the center of your pelvis as the accordion closes inwardly.

DURATION:

Thirty to sixty seconds.

6. *The Hammock*

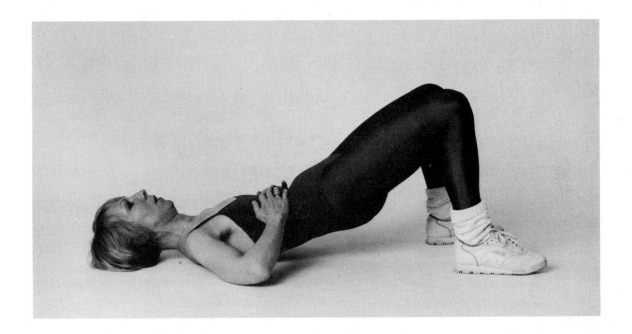

POSITION:	Lie supine, with your knees bent and your feet flat on the floor.
ACTIVITY:	Inhale, and then exhale as you slowly raise your hips up toward the ceiling. Inhale and then exhale while slowly lowering your hips back down to the floor.
IMAGE:	Imagine that the inhalation begins at your pelvis and travels up your back. See your back opening and widening out to the sides. The exhale passes your lips, your chin, your sternum, and your rib cage and drops down into your abdominals as you raise your hips upward. Use the same image for breathing as you lower the hips to the floor.
REPETITIONS:	Four.

7. *Transverse Abdominals*
(FIRST AND SECOND TRIMESTERS AND POSTPARTUM)

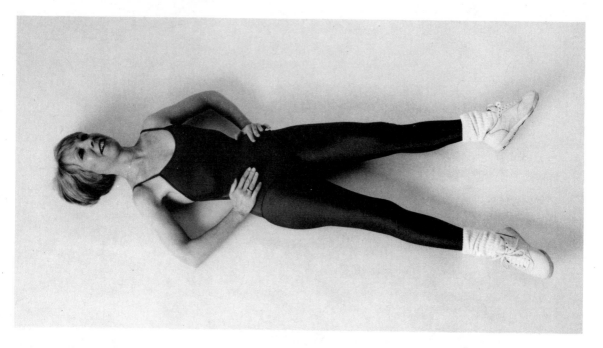

POSITION:

Lie supine, with your legs long. Place your hands on your hipbones.

ACTIVITY:

Inhale, and then exhale as you press your hipbones in toward your belly button, causing your legs to rotate inwardly. Feel your lower back flatten on the floor as your abdominals press down toward your spine. Inhale, and then exhale as you allow the hipbones to return to their neutral position as your legs rotate outwardly.

IMAGE:

As your hipbones move from their neutral position toward your belly button on the exhale, imagine that an eye is placed on top of each hipbone and that the eyes turn toward each other so that they can "see" each other. The "eyes" return to their normal position on the inhale.

REPETITIONS:

Five to ten.

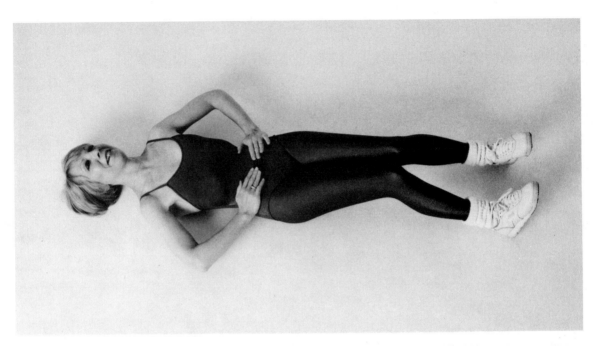

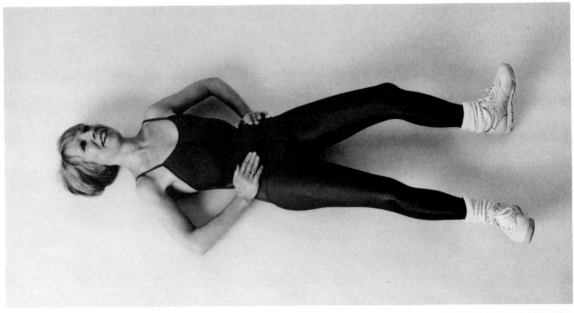

8. Forward Curl-up, Arms Reach Forward

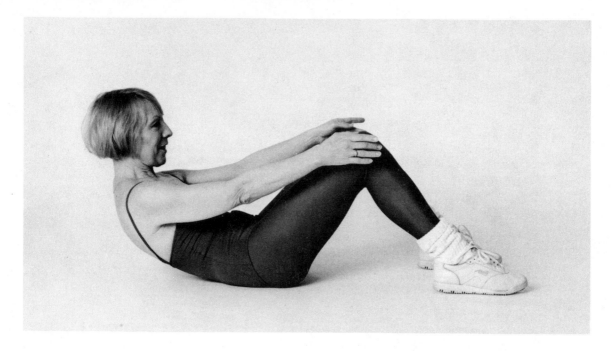

POSITION:

Lie supine, with your knees bent and your feet flat on the floor.

ACTIVITY:

Inhale, and then exhale as you tilt your pelvis down and press your abdominals to the floor, allowing your head and shoulders to come off the floor. Reach your hands toward your knees. Concentrate on pressing your belly button to the ground.

REPETITIONS:

Ten to twenty.

9. *Diagonal Curl-up, Arms Reach Forward*

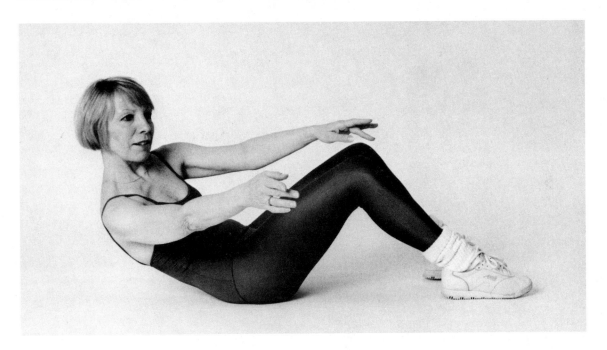

POSITION: Lie supine, with your knees bent and your feet flat on the floor.

ACTIVITY: Inhale, and then exhale as you tilt your pelvis to the floor. Press your abdominals downward while allowing your head to come up and your left hand to reach toward your right knee with your arms extended and parallel. Keep your belly button pressed to the floor.

REPETITIONS: Ten with right diagonal twist; ten with left diagonal twist.

10. *Repeat: Psoa Racer's Stretch*

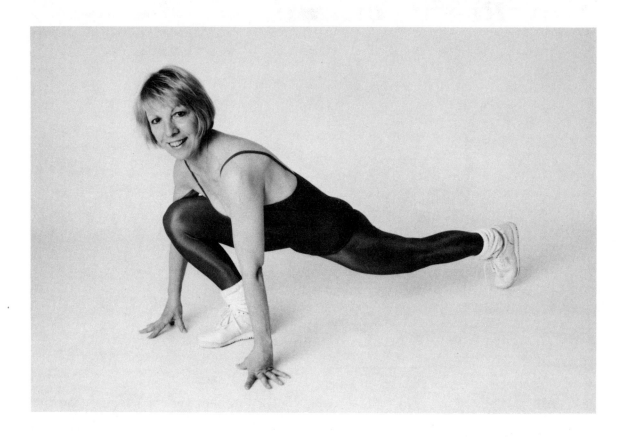

POSITION: Lunge forward on your right leg, and extend your left leg behind you. Keep your right knee over your right foot.

ACTIVITY: Stretch your left hip down toward the floor.

IMAGE: See your left hip stretching and lengthening like a rubber band.

DURATION: Thirty to sixty seconds. Repeat with other leg.

Prenatal Exercise

SECOND TRIMESTER

1. *Cheerleader Stretch*
2. *Pelvic Floor Exercise*
3. *Deep Abdominal Breathing While Lying on the Left Side*
4. *Pelvic Tilt in Supine Position*
5. *Pelvic Tilt with Legs Long and Knees Soft*
6. *The Hammock*
7. *Transverse Abdominals*
8. *Forward Curl-up, with Arms Crossed*
9. *Diagonal Curl-up, with Arms Crossed*
10. *Repeat: Cheerleader Stretch*

1. *Cheerleader Stretch*

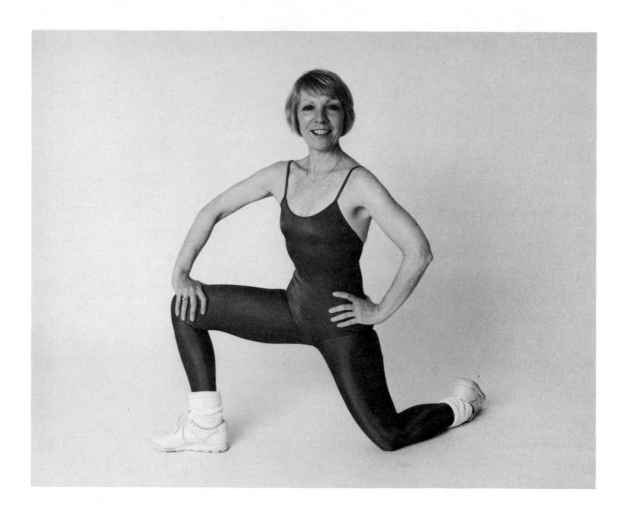

POSITION: Kneel on your left knee with your right foot flat on the floor.

ACTIVITY: Push gently and stretch your left hip forward, with your right hand on your right knee for support. Then place both elbows on your right knee and lean forward.

IMAGE: Breathe into your left hip, and imagine it expanding and opening like a beam of light.

DURATION: Thirty to sixty seconds.

Repeat with the other leg

2. *Pelvic Floor Exercise*
(DURING ENTIRE PREGNANCY AND POSTPARTUM)

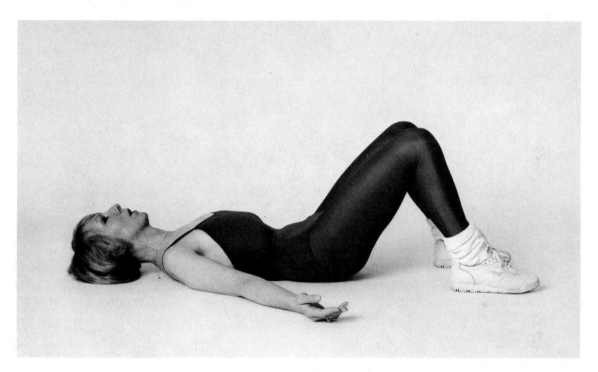

POSITION:	Lie supine, with your knees bent and your feet flat on the floor, or sit comfortably in any position.
ACTIVITY:	You should feel several muscle groups working together— your bladder, rectum and vagina (called the perineum). Contract and squeeze the perineum together. (It should feel as though you are trying to stop or control urination.) Release and let go.
IMAGE:	Think of "lifting from within and pulling up to your center." Release the innermost spaces first and then the perineum.
REPETITIONS:	Twenty to fifty.
NOTE:	After you have gained proficiency, hold for a count of five and release. Repeat ten to twenty times.

3. Deep Abdominal Breathing While Lying on the Left Side

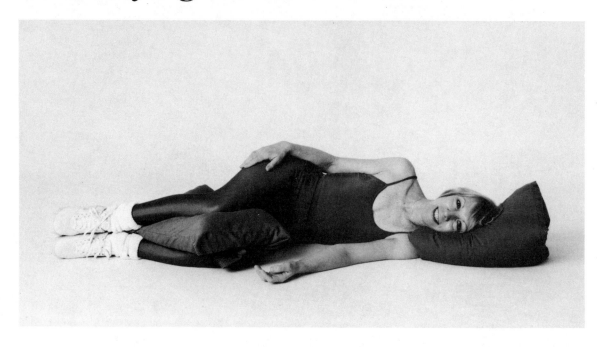

POSITION: Lie on your left side with your knees bent in front of you and separated by a pillow. Support your head with a pillow. Place your hands on your abdominal area.

ACTIVITY: Inhaling through your nose, feel your tummy expand three-dimensionally. Continue your inhalation, slowly and deeply. Don't rush it to avoid getting dizzy. When you feel ready to exhale, allow your lips to part slightly and let the breath pass your lips, chin, collarbone, sternum, rib cage, diaphragm, and all the way down to the abdominal area. Repeat this process several times.

IMAGE: Imagine your breath encompassing and gently caressing your baby.

DURATION: Three to five minutes.

4. *Pelvic Tilt in Supine Position*

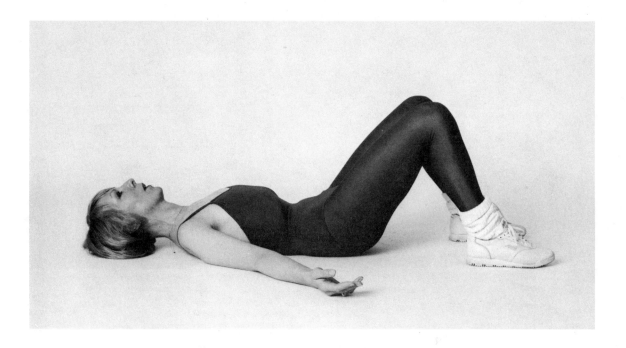

POSITION:	Lie supine, with your knees bent and your feet flat on the floor.
ACTIVITY:	Inhale, and then exhale as you pull your abdomen in toward your spine while flattening the spine against the floor.
IMAGE:	Imagine that your belly button is a vortex, where a swirling mass of water drains down to the floor.
REPETITIONS:	Ten.

5. *Pelvic Tilt with Legs Long and Knees Soft*

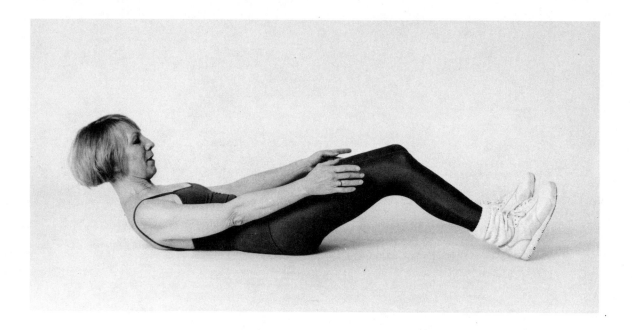

POSITION:

Lie supine with your knees bent and your feet flat on the floor.

ACTIVITY:

1. Inhale. As you exhale, press your abdominals down to the floor as you stretch your legs long underneath you. Try to keep your lower back pressed to the floor as long as you can.

2. Inhale. As you exhale, press your abdominals down to the floor and bend your knees and ankles slightly. Raise your head, neck, and shoulders off the floor. Repeat several times.

IMAGE:

On the inhalation, see the spine and legs stretching away from each other in opposite directions just like an accordion. On the exhalation, see the energy of the spine and legs converging to the center of your pelvis as the accordion closes inwardly.

DURATION:

Thirty to sixty seconds.

6. *The Hammock*

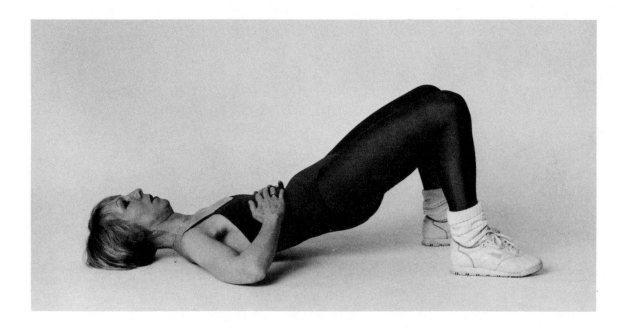

POSITION: Lie supine, with your knees bent and your feet flat on the floor.

ACTIVITY: Inhale, and then exhale slowly as you raise your hips up toward the ceiling. Inhale and then exhale while slowly lowering your hips back down to the floor.

IMAGE: Imagine that the inhalation begins at your pelvis and travels up your back. See your back opening and widening out to the sides. The exhale passes your lips, your chin, your sternum, and your rib cage and drops down into your abdominals as you raise your hips upward. Use the same image for breathing as you lower the hips to the floor.

REPETITIONS: Four.

7. *Transverse Abdominals*

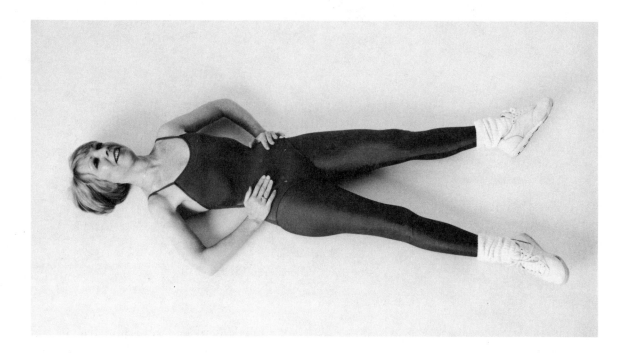

POSITION:

Lie supine, with your legs long. Place your hands on your hipbones.

ACTIVITY:

Inhale, and then exhale as you press your hipbones in toward your belly button, causing your legs to rotate inwardly. Feel your lower back flatten on the floor as your abdominals press down toward your spine. Inhale, and then exhale as you allow the hipbones to return to their neutral position.

IMAGE:

As your hipbones move from their neutral position toward your belly button on the exhale, imagine that an eye is placed on top of each hipbone and that the eyes turn toward each other so that they can "see" each other. The "eyes" return to their normal position on the inhale.

REPETITIONS:

Five to ten.

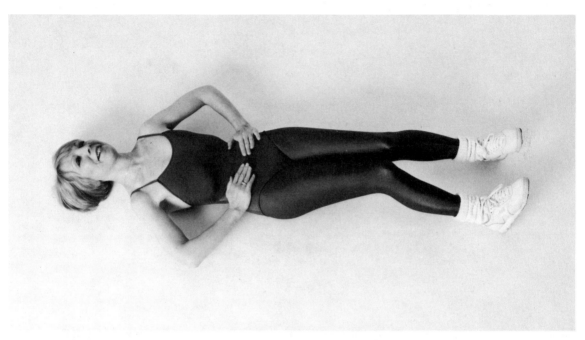

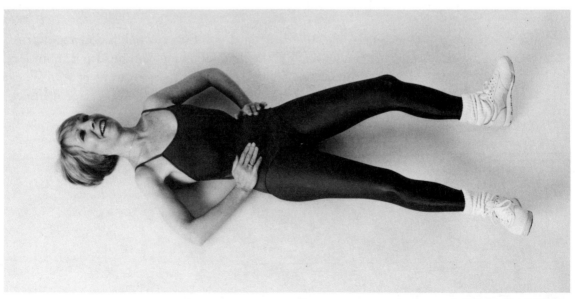

8. Forward Curl-up, with Arms Crossed

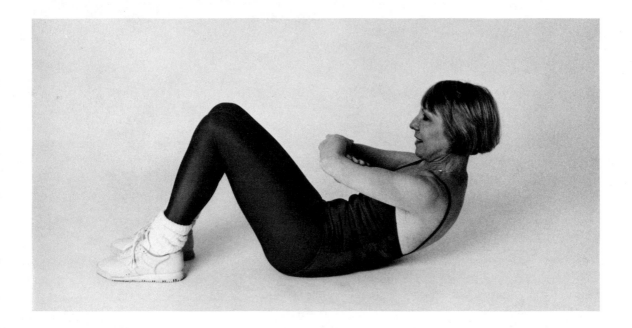

POSITION:

Lie supine, with your knees bent and your feet flat on the floor.

ACTIVITY:

Inhale, and then exhale as you tilt your pelvis down and press your abdominals to the floor, allowing your head and shoulders to come off the floor. Cross your arms in front of your chest with each hand grasping the opposite elbow. Concentrate on pressing your belly button to the ground.

REPETITIONS:

Ten to twenty.

9. *Diagonal Curl-up, with Crossed Arms*

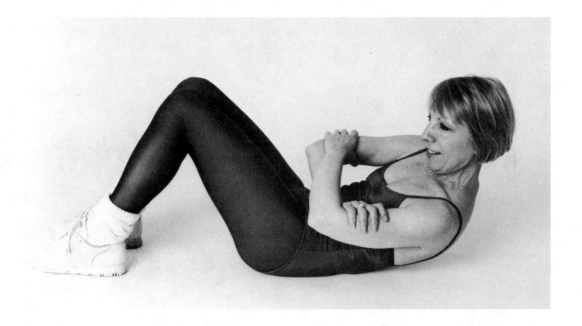

POSITION: Lie supine, with your knees bent and your feet flat on the floor.

ACTIVITY: Inhale, and then exhale as you tilt your pelvis to the floor. Press your abdominals downward, allowing your head to come up and your right shoulder to reach toward your left knee, with your arms crossed in front of your chest. Keep your belly button pressed to the floor.

REPETITIONS: Ten with right diagonal twist; ten with left diagonal twist.

10. *Repeat: Cheerleader Stretch*

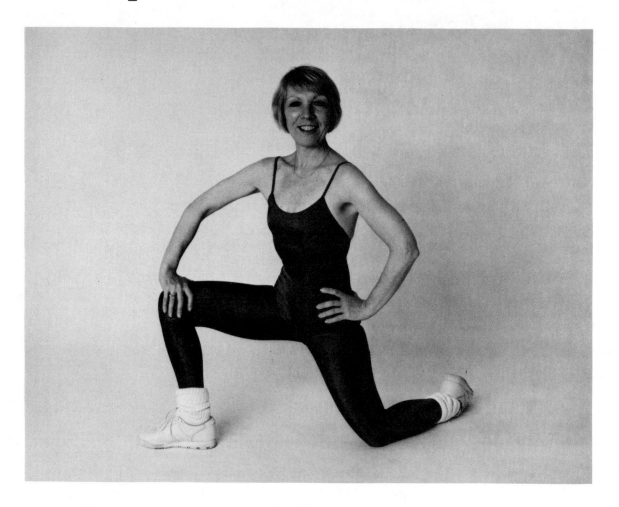

POSITION: Kneel on your left knee with your right foot flat on the floor.

ACTIVITY: Push gently and stretch your left hip forward with your right hand on your right knee for support. Then place both elbows on your right knee and lean forward.

IMAGE: Breathe into your left hip, and imagine it expanding and opening like a beam of light.

DURATION: Thirty to sixty seconds.

Repeat with the other leg.

Prenatal Exercise

THIRD TRIMESTER

1. *Chair Stretch for the Psoas*
2. *Pelvic Floor Exercise*
3. *Centered Deep Breathing*
4. *Pelvic Tilt from All Fours*
5. *Pelvic Tilt with Back Against a Wall*
6. *Pelvic Pull Under*
7. *Backward Curl-down*
8. *Diagonal Curl-down*
9. *Repeat: Chair Stretch for the Psoas*

1. *Chair Stretch for the Psoas*
(THIRD TRIMESTER)

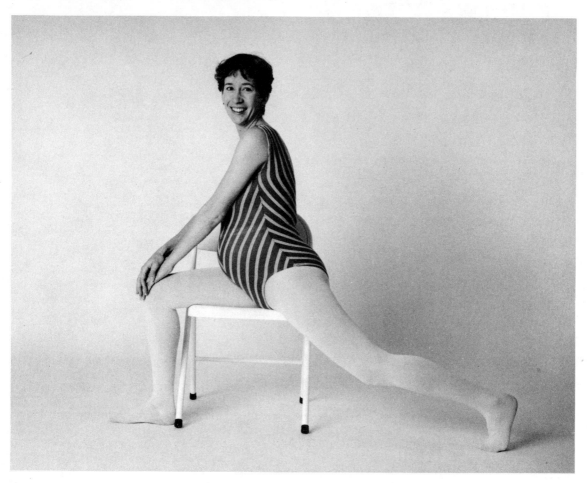

POSITION:	Sit sideways on a chair on your right hip with your left leg behind you, and your hands on your right knee.
ACTIVITY:	Stretch your left leg behind you as far as you can, as you press your left hip forward.
IMAGE:	Imagine that you have a wheel at the level of your hip joint that is rotating in a clockwise direction as the energy of the leg extends behind you.
DURATION:	Thirty to sixty seconds.

2. *Pelvic Floor Exercise*
(DURING ENTIRE PREGNANCY AND POSTPARTUM)

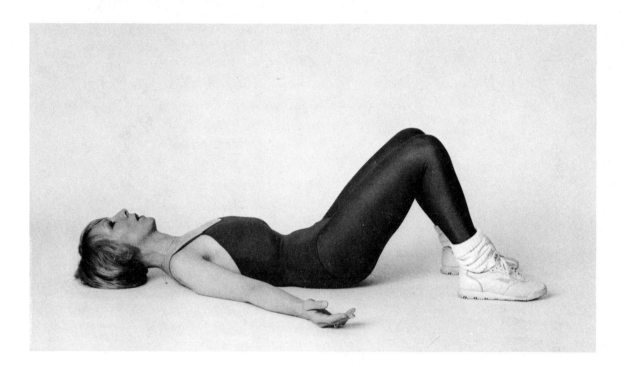

POSITION:	Lie supine, with your knees bent and your feet flat on the floor, or sit comfortably in any position.
ACTIVITY:	You should feel several muscle groups working together—your bladder, rectum, and vagina (called the perineum). Contract and squeeze the perineum together. (It should feel as though you are trying to stop or control urination.) Release and let go.
IMAGE:	Think of "lifting from within and pulling up to your center." Release the innermost spaces first and then the perineum.
REPETITIONS:	Twenty to fifty.
NOTE:	After you have gained proficiency, hold for a count of five and release. Repeat ten to twenty times.

3. Centered Deep Breathing

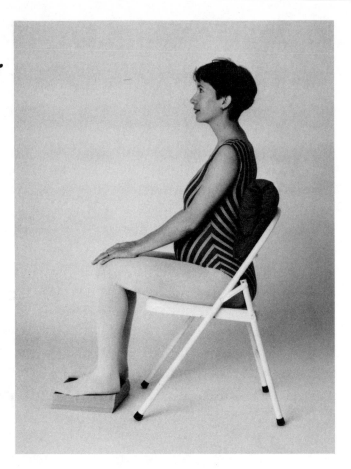

POSITION: Sit on a chair with a straight back. Place your pelvis directly against the back of the chair, using a cushion if it makes you more comfortable. Feel yourself balanced on your two "sitz bones." Your knees should be bent and slightly higher than your thighs with your feet flat on the floor. (If your feet don't touch the floor, place them on top of a telephone book.) Rest your hands comfortably on your thighs.

ACTIVITY: Breathe naturally; inhale through your nose and exhale through your mouth. Repeat several times.

IMAGE: Imagine your spine to be a long thermometer. See the thermometer's red mercury travel up your spine on the inhale and slide down your spine on the exhale.

DURATION: Three to five minutes.

4. Pelvic Tilt from All Fours

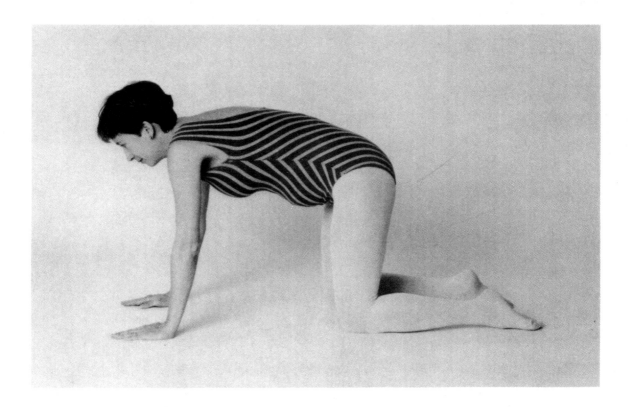

POSITION: Get down on all fours, making sure your knees are under your hips and your wrists are under your shoulders. Keep your back flat in its neutral position, with your head in line with your spine. Your arms and legs should not move.

ACTIVITY: Pull your abdominal muscles toward your spine and press up to the ceiling with your lower back, rounding your back slightly. Hold for the count of ten. Release to the neutral position. Repeat several times.

IMAGE: Imagine that you are a cat rounding your back in a stretch.

DURATION: Thirty to sixty seconds.

5. Pelvic Tilt with Back Against a Wall

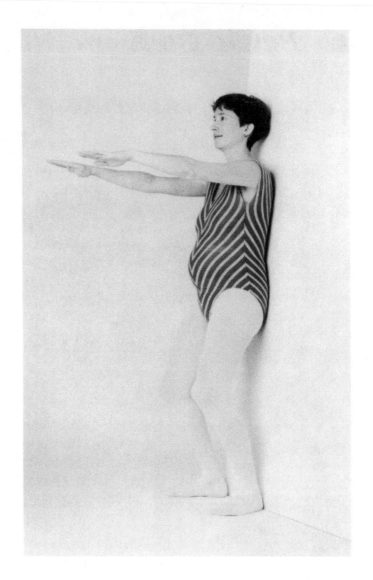

POSITION: Stand with your back against a wall in the neutral (natural curve) position.

ACTIVITY: Bend your knees and slide down the wall with your back. Gently press your lower back to the wall. Stay in this position for the count of ten. Repeat several times.

IMAGE: As you bend your knees and slide downward, see your tummy being uplifted as though it was at the top end of a seesaw.

DURATION: Thirty to sixty seconds.

6. *Pelvic Pull Under*

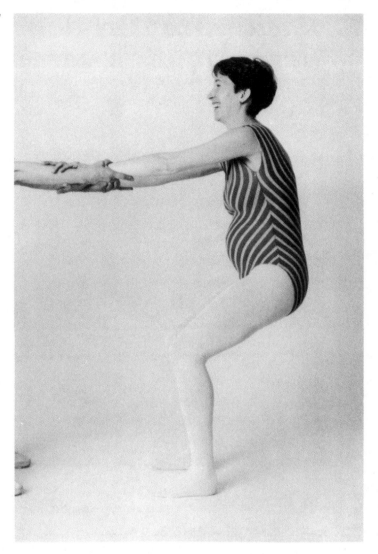

POSITION: Kneel or stand while holding onto a very secure object such as a doorway or another person as demonstrated here.

ACTIVITY: Pull away from your partner or the stationary object, and exhale as you round your lower back, pulling your abdominal muscles in toward your spine.

IMAGE: See yourself as taffy being gently pulled and stretched.

DURATION: Thirty to sixty seconds.

7. Backward Curl-down
(THIRD TRIMESTER AND POSTPARTUM)

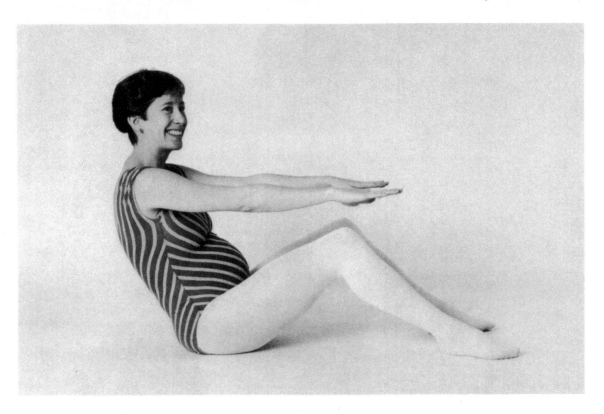

POSITION: Begin sitting upright, hands reaching toward your knees.

ACTIVITY: Round your lower spine under and lean back as far as you can without falling down, then slowly return upright.

IMAGE: See your belly button being pulled to the floor.

REPETITIONS: Ten to twenty.

8. *Diagonal Curl-down*
(THIRD TRIMESTER AND POSTPARTUM)

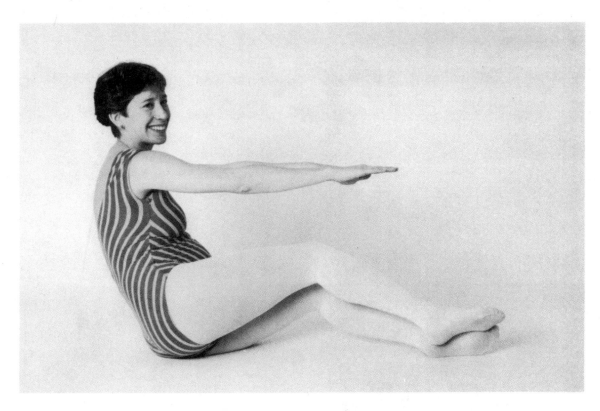

POSITION:	Begin sitting upright, with your weight shifted onto your left hip and your right hip off the floor; your hands reaching forward toward your right knee.
ACTIVITY:	Round your lower spine under and lean back as far as you can without falling down, then slowly return to the upright position.
IMAGE:	See your belly button being pulled to the floor.
REPETITIONS:	Ten to twenty with weight on left hip; ten to twenty on opposite side.

9. Repeat: Chair Stretch for the Psoas

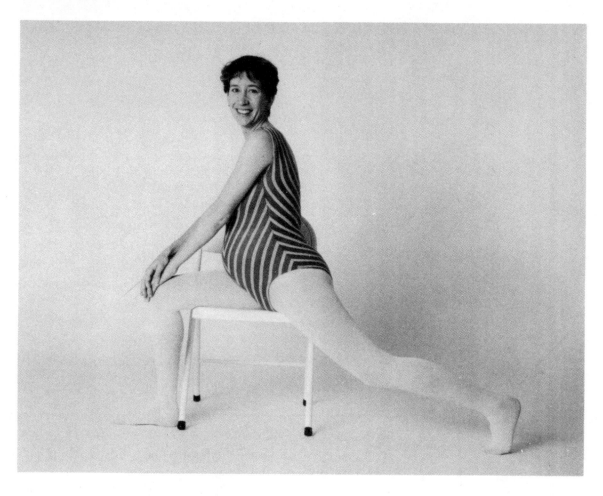

POSITION: Sit sideways on a chair on your right hip with your left leg behind you, and your hands on your right knee.

ACTIVITY: Stretch your left leg behind you as far as you can, as you press your left hip forward.

IMAGE: Imagine that you have a wheel at the level of your hip joint that is rotating in a counterclockwise direction as the energy of the leg extends behind you.

DURATION: Thirty to sixty seconds.

POSTPARTUM EXERCISE

After you've had your baby, you'll want to restore your body as quickly as possible to the state of efficiency and fitness that existed before pregnancy. Physiological changes will occur immediately, and exercising will show results in days. Because of hormonal changes, however, your joints will remain vulnerable to injury for several weeks. For this reason, maintaining good postural habits is essential until the hormone levels return to normal and the muscles regain their former length and strength.

The first order of the day will be to stretch the psoas and strengthen the abdominal wall to realign the pelvis in its correct relationship to the spine. It is imperative, however, that you bring the muscles of the pelvic floor back to tone before embarking on a path of strenuous abdominal exercises. If you do strenuous abdominal exercises before the pelvic floor is in condition, there is a much greater tendency toward bladder incontinence. Therefore, the abdominal exercises listed below are mild to moderate.

Remember, weakened muscles can make you susceptible to injury or the development of back pain from the least cause. You can begin your postpartum exercises as early as twenty-four hours after giving birth, but consult with your physician before you start. The beginning exercise sessions should be done often for short periods of time, not for long, tiring sessions. You will have to build slowly and gradually to a real workout.

You will need to correct the postpartum pelvic tilt as well. I've had many women come to my classes after giving birth who say, "No matter what I do, I can't seem to flatten my tummy. I always seem to have this bulge." My response to them usually is, "Well, if the bulge is subcutaneous fat, it will burn off when you exercise aerobically. However, it is probably the result of a shortened, tightened psoas, which is preventing the correct placement of the pelvis and proper strengthening of all the fibers of the abdominals." I then proceed to give them psoas stretches and abdominal strengtheners, which I will now give to you.

Postpartum Exercises

1. Psoas Stretch:
   Start with the Stretch for a Stubborn Psoas (p. 165). When you begin to feel progress in your flexibility, start doing other psoas stretches.
2. Pelvic Floor
3. Deep Breathing
4. Pelvic Tilt in Supine Position
5. Pelvic Tilt with Legs Long and Knees Soft
6. The Hammock
7. Transverse Abdominals
8. Backward Curl-down
9. Diagonal Curl-down
10. Forward Curl-up with Crossed Arms
11. Diagonal Curl-up with Crossed Arms
12. Psoas Stretch: Any variation

Postpartum Tips

The exercises presented in this book can be modified to your individual level of prior training, level of tolerance, and your labor and delivery experience.

1. Stretch your psoas so that your pelvis can be realigned to prevent backache and so that you can strengthen your abdominals effectively. Exercises for the psoas are on pages 188, 200, and 212.
2. Check for separation of the abdominals. This is when the muscles separate due to the trauma of birth. It may take a while for the muscles to heal and for the fibers to interdigitate again. Perform the simple abdominal curl-up with your hands on the abdominal area. If you feel a separation (when the abdominals have not rejoined) of more than two or three fingers, do not do the abdominal exercises. Go back to pelvic floor exercises and try curl-downs.
3. Make allowances for weakness in your pelvic floor or abdominal wall. Don't follow the suggested repetitions if an exercise feels particularly difficult for you. Use your own judgment, and listen to what your body tells you.
4. The postpartum exercise sequence should be:
   A. Stretch your psoas.

B. Strengthen the pelvic floor.

C. Strengthen the abdominals in the neutral position.

D. Strengthen the abdominals in the diagonal or oblique position.

5. If the rectus abdominus muscles have separated, it is important for them to heal before doing oblique abdominal exercises. If this is the case, perform only the forward curl-downs in the neutral position or the forward curl-ups in the neutral position.

6. Gradually increase the difficulty and the repetitions as you become stronger.

7. In addition to the exercises presented in this book for the psoas, lower back, pelvic floor, and abdominals, you should engage in some regular aerobic activity to burn fat. (See Chapter 5.)

LIFTING AND CARRYING BABIES AND CHILDREN

- If your baby is lying in a bassinet that is too low for you to reach down and pick him or her up without strain, make sure you bend your knees and place one foot ahead of the other before you reach down. Or if your back is particularly bothersome, place a chair next to the bassinet, sit down, pick up your baby, and then come up to standing. The same would hold true for a crib with a collapsible side.

- Picking up your baby from a kneeling position will help prevent strain on your back. Select a playpen with sides that can fold down for this purpose.

- If you don't have a changing table that is the proper height, kneel down and change your baby on the floor.

- Avoid carrying the baby on one hip. Straddle the baby's legs in front of you around both your hips, or carry the baby on your back or against your chest in a carrier designed specifically for that purpose.

- If you are giving your child a top-of-the-shoulders piggyback ride, don't swing him or her up from a standing position. Have your child climb up onto a chair and then onto a table; then place your back to the table and rest your buttocks on the table. Then let your child climb up onto your shoulders.

Shift yourself forward off the table while keeping your knees bent. Slowly straighten your knees up to vertical.

- If you are an urban dweller and have to carry a stroller with your baby in it up or down the subway stairs, get someone to help you. If that is impossible, bend your knees grabbing the stroller closest to its center of gravity, and bring it as close to your body as you can so that you can spread the distribution of weight.

7

Musculoskeletal Injuries and Treatment

"Oh, my aching back" is the cry of approximately 80 percent of our population. Some pains can be irksome at best and debilitating at worst. Once the pain sets in, it's important to pinpoint the cause. It might be a slight muscle pull, or it could be a more severe tear of the muscle fibers. These kinds of injuries are usually very localized and are tender, swollen, or knotted. They can be relieved relatively quickly with ice and rest. Less easy to identify, however, are more complex back afflictions and serious pathological (disease-related) conditions, which should be properly diagnosed by a physician.

SERIOUS BACK CONDITIONS

Since it is not the purpose of this book to offer treatment for serious pathological conditions, I will simply describe some of the more common disorders and then refer you to the Suggested Reading section for books that deal more completely with these conditions. I will limit myself to the pathological conditions of herniated disk, sciatica, and scoliosis. If any of the symptoms described apply to you, see your physician immediately.

Herniated Disk/Sciatica

As mentioned in Chapter 1, the bony segments of the spine or vertebrae are cushioned from each other with soft, jellylike tissue called disks. In a normal back each disk remains contained between the sections of bone that it supports and cushions. However, chronic misuse or injury can cause a disk to bulge out from between the vertebrae. A bulging disk, sometimes called a "slipped disk," may press on a nerve emanating from the spine. When this occurs, a person often experiences pain shooting down one or both legs and sometimes numbness or tingling in the foot. This is usually referred to as sciatica, and it is a "must" to consult your physician.

If you have a herniated or torn disk, it is reassuring to know that 85 percent of your fellow sufferers respond to conservative treatment, which would include rest, appropriate medication, and moderate stretching and extension movements rather than surgery. Exercise is crucial for recovery, but consult your physician before starting such a program.

Scoliosis

Scoliosis is a lateral (sideways) bending curve of the spine, which usually causes one hip to be higher than the other and the opposite shoulder to be higher than the other (for example, the right hip high, with the left shoulder high). The cause may be congenital (one that you are born with), in which case the skeletal structure cannot be changed. Or it can be functional (without a known organic cause), evolving as a result of improper usage of the body and poor postural habits. In this case, although not fully correctable, ameliorating changes can occur in the skeletal structure with gentle movements and stretching exercises of the psoas.

Another condition affecting the lateral curve of the spine is a difference in leg length, which will cause compensatory changes in the spine. This condition can be helped with an orthotic (shoe lift) to correct improper use of the limbs and to retrain the legs for more efficient movement and postural habits.

A shortened psoas can pull the spine into a scoliotic condition. This can be corrected provided new neuromuscular patterns and proper postural habits are learned.

Referred Back Pain	The reader should be aware that lower back pain can be *referred* from other systems such as the kidneys, female reproductive organs, gastrointestinal tract, and pancreas and that it can arise from various diseases of the muscle and the peripheral and central nervous systems. The diagnosis of these conditions is beyond the scope of this book. But their possibility must not be forgotten, and examinations and tests must be performed to rule them out. Exercise can help to alleviate symptoms, but the real pathology must be treated by a physician for permanent relief to occur.

LESS SERIOUS BACK INJURIES AND THEIR TREATMENT

What Can Be Injured	**Muscle** injuries occur when the muscle fibers are torn. Because the muscles have an ample blood supply, they usually repair quickly and easily within a few days.

Tendons, which attach the muscles to the bones, are made of tough fibrous material that is fairly inelastic. Their blood supply is very limited, and they take longer to heal if injured.

Often as tendons heal, extraneous internal scar tissue forms. Normal scar tissue production is an important part of healing, but abnormal scarring tends to keep retearing through usage, creating a cycle of reinjury. Abnormal scar tissue forms during the enforced rest caused by the injury, and when activity is resumed and the tissue tears again, it is called tendinitis. Gentle stretching exercises following an injury will prevent excessive scar tissue from forming and make the area less vulnerable to reinjury.

Ligaments attach bones to each other and are made of tough material, like tendons, but are even more inelastic because their blood supply is very limited. Their primary function is to stabilize the joints and prevent abnormal movements and dislocations. Depending on the severity of the injury, ligaments can take anywhere from six weeks to a year to heal.

Cartilage is a soft fibrous material that acts as a shock absorber and smooth, gliding surface between bones. It has a limited blood supply, and when it heals at all, it does so slowly and poorly. A slipped disk is cartilage that has moved from its place between the vertebrae.

Nerves are the communication wires in our bodies. When some part of a nerve is pinched or pressed upon, there can be intense pain, weakness, numbness, or a feeling of pins and needles in the area supplied by that nerve. Nerve pressure can cause referred pain from great distances. Sciatic pain down the back of the leg is caused by pressure on the sciatic nerve, which is in the pelvic area.

What Causes Back Injury?

1. Poor alignment of the bones can cause injuries, especially near the joints.
2. Chronic muscle tension will leave your body less supple and less able to absorb the shocks and stresses of moving. Muscles that are tight and rigid cannot warm up or stretch easily. Chronic tension means that your muscle fibers are in a state of contraction.
3. Lack of sufficient stretch can lead to tears of all kinds. If your muscles are well stretched out, they have the extra give that can protect you. Stretching when you are cold or stretching incorrectly by bouncing ballistically can tear your muscles or tendons.
4. Muscle imbalance can be destructive. When one muscle group is strong and another muscle group is relatively weak, it can create an uneven workload and can throw off the alignment at the joints.
5. Fatigue frequently precedes injury. A tired muscle will not be able to respond to extra stress. The reflexes are slower, and the likelihood of injury is greatly increased.
6. Knowing the limits of your strength is essential to avoid injury. If you try to use a muscle beyond its capacity, particularly when fatigued, it will become vulnerable to injury. Often taxing a muscle beyond its capacity can actually erode your strength. Minimal exertion beyond your previous limit builds strength. Attempts at too rapid a progression can result in damaged tissue and increased

tension. One extra repetition may increase your strength, but ten more may give you a back spasm.

7. Exercising without a proper warm-up can often lead to muscle and tendon injuries. Cold muscles are stiff and easily pulled or torn. When muscles are properly warmed up, they are more pliable, stretch farther, contract more vigorously and quickly, and are less prone to strain and other injuries.

8. Performing exercise in a class too advanced for you pushes your body too quickly. To continue in such a class could be a tragic mistake that results in torn muscles and inflamed tendons. Exercise at your level of skill, and progress slowly.

Types of Back Injuries

Diffuse Muscle Pain

The most common cause of short-term muscle pain is usually a viral systemic infection, which subsides with medical treatment. Long-term chronic diffuse muscle aching is usually related to deconditioning, degenerative arthritis with secondary muscular effects, or to psychological factors. An exercise program for diffuse back muscle pain would be beneficial for reconditioning, increasing range of motion, and as a form of stress reduction.

Muscle Spasm

A muscle spasm is a sudden contraction of a muscle that causes it to knot up. The most common cause of muscle spasm is performing an activity that is excessive for the condition of the muscle. This often occurs when muscles have not been sufficiently warmed up. Usually the spasm will release after being stretched.

Whenever you injure a muscle, swelling occurs to prevent further movement that could cause further injury. Without movement, muscles atrophy and weaken. Therefore, if you have an injury-related spasm with accompanying inflammation, use ice to reduce the swelling and to relieve the spasm. However, if the muscle spasm is not caused by an injury, it can be treated with moist heat, which will release the spasm but will increase any inflammation.

Acute Sprain

Sprain results in the tearing of ligaments. Sprain can be acute or chronic. Acute sprain usually follows an injury, as a result of a sudden force for which the muscle was not prepared. The higher the proportion of fibers torn, the more severe the tear and pain will be. In the case of back sprain, the pain is usually severe, spread over the lower back, and is associated with muscle spasm. Any motion is painful and will aggravate the spasm.

If you suffer acute lower back pain, lie down on a hard mattress or the floor with one or two cushions placed behind your knees and a rolled towel placed under the base of your skull. Do centered deep breathing (pages 36–38). Light massage can be helpful, but deep massage and manipulation are not recommended. As the pain subsides and you have regained full range of motion, you should start an exercise program to stretch out contracted muscles gradually and restore motion and strength. Be sure your back is completely healed before you begin, so you won't be vulnerable to reinjury.

Chronic Strain

Strain due to overexertion results in torn muscle fibers accompanied by a slight swelling or inflammation. This syndrome is probably the most common lower back condition. In its milder form it can be experienced as a lower backache that is improved by rest but aggravated by bending or lifting. Rarely is the pain severe for long periods of time. As the severity increases, muscle spasm occurs in response to movement, restriction of range of motion, and abnormal postural compensations. In severe cases a period of rest may be indicated as described for acute lower back sprain. If you suffer from chronic lower back strain, it is essential that you perform stretching and strengthening exercises and learn proper postural principles for sleeping, sitting, and efficient body mechanics (see Chapter 8).

Chronic strains are caused by insufficient muscle flexibility or an imbalance between the strength of opposing muscles. The following are classifications of strain and sprain in order of least severity.

- First-degree strain: an overstretched muscle with possible slight tearing.
- Second-degree strain: a partial or more extensive tear.
- Third-degree sprain: a complete ligimentous or muscular tear.

First-degree and mild second-degree strains should be treated with Rest, Ice, Compression, and Elevation (RICE). With rest, a strain will heal in a few days. Stretching exercises should be done to help prevent recurrence.

Stretching exercises are equally as important when dealing with chronic strains. Strengthening the muscle in relation to its opposing muscle is also recommended.

Third-degree sprains should be referred to an orthopedist.

Bed Rest

If your back pain is severe, you may require complete bed rest. If the pain is due to a spasm, the vicious cycle must be broken. The spasm functions as a kind of splint that causes the muscles to go into contraction to reduce the motion of an injured area. The more you move, the more the muscle spasms, resulting in greater pain. With bed rest, the possibility of motion is reduced and therefore the muscles can relax. However, muscles become weak and deconditioned very quickly, and so the period of bed rest should be limited to three to five days, if possible.

Once your contracted muscles have released sufficiently and you can move about, begin doing movements that involve changing body positions. Move from lying down to sitting. If any of the movements cause pain, stop the activity and rest.

Recovery Exercises Following Lower Back Muscle Strain

Lying Down:
1. Do gentle stretching movements of your arms, legs, and torso.
2. Gently pull your abdominal muscles in toward your spine, and tilt your pelvis back toward the floor or bed. Roll to your side and come up to sitting.

Sitting:
1. Drop your head and roll your spine down until your chin

is resting on your knees with your hands on your thighs. Stay here and breathe.

2. To recover, shift your pelvis back and push up with your hands. Slowly roll your spine up to vertical.

Sex and the Bad Back
Generally speaking, a person with back problems should not be concerned that sex will cause pain or permanent damage to the back. However, consult with your physician if you fall into the two following major areas of concern: (1) if you have a serious disease or infection, tumor, or inflammatory arthritis or (2) if you have significant or "true" instability of the back with potential for neurological impairment (for example, paralysis of the lower extremity or bladder function).

If you have back pain while making love, use common sense and adjust your posture accordingly. The task is simply to find some way to satisfy both the person with back pain and the partner. It is usually better for the symptomatic patient to be more passive.

Sexual activity when acute back pain has subsided can be viewed as a rehabilitative exercise that can help overcome the back problem and minimize attacks in the future. The basic movement for the sex act is the pelvic thrust, which is the same as the pelvic tilt. It involves the same muscles that must be strengthened to prevent chronic back pain—the lower abdominals contract and the muscles of the low back stretch. Therefore, it can be said that sexual intercourse is a first-rate exercise for backache prevention!

8

Changing Your Everyday Habits for a Healthier Back

Time and thought given to proper body mechanics bring the rewards of safer, easier daily movement and the elimination of muscular aches and pains. If you learn to use proper body mechanics in your everyday activities, you can reduce muscular work and its accompanying strain, eliminate inefficient motion, increase safety of movement, and convey a sense of ease and grace. Backache will invariably result from continued poor body mechanics in everyday movement. Replacing back-damaging habits with back-sparing habits along with performing stretching and strengthening exercises should be the basis of your prevention program.

> *Myth:* Since strong muscles prevent injury, strengthening exercises for the back will prevent pain and injury.
>
> *Correction:* It is not strong back muscles that prevent back injury, but muscles that are flexible and well balanced in terms of strength.

SITTING

> *Myth:* Sitting rests the back.

Correction: Sitting is more stressful to disks in the lumbar spine than standing or bending forward. The best way to sit is on a firm chair with a back rest, placing a pillow in the small of the back and using some form of support under the feet.

A back's best friend is a hard, straightback chair. If you can't get the chair you prefer, learn how to sit properly on whatever chair you have.

Try to use a straightback chair that supports both your upper and lower back. The seat of the chair should be firm and low enough for your feet to rest entirely on the floor. If your legs are short, place some form of support under your feet to raise your knees above your hips.

The support for the back should be behind the pelvis, not at the center of the back. When the pelvis is placed against the back of the chair, there is less of an opportunity to shift your weight back on to the tailbone. If the seat is too deep, place a firm pillow between the back of the chair and your lower back for support. You should feel your weight placed equally on both "sitz-bones."

If you must sit for long periods of time, try to move around and change positions. Stand up from time to time to stretch and give yourself a break.

Sitting at a Desk

Use a rolling office chair with lumbar support. Keep the chair close enough to the working surface so that you bend your torso forward at the thigh joints rather than from the spine. Keep both feet flat on the floor to give stability to the pelvis.

To Sit Down

Stand close to the chair. Place one foot close to or just under the chair. Bend the trunk forward at the thigh joints, *never at the waist*. Aim your buttocks toward the chair, and let your legs control the movement of your body weight. If you need the assistance of your arms, place your hands on the arms or sides of the chair seat, and slowly lower your body down to the chair.

To Stand

Reverse the motion described above to come up to standing. Rock your torso forward at the hip joint. Shift the weight of your body onto your feet as you lean forward. Slowly drop your tailbone down as you straighten up through your thighs. Feel your spine lengthen into the upright position.

DRIVING

When driving, move your car seat as close to the wheel as you can. It should be far enough forward so that your knees are slightly higher than your hips. If the seat is too deep, use pillows to give your lower and middle back support. Try to operate the accelerator and brake with just your foot and not your whole leg. Try to avoid sitting for longer than a half hour at a stretch. Take a rest break. Get out of the car. Move and stretch.

STANDING

Myth: The proper way to stand is with the heels turned out.

Correction: The proper way to stand is with the feet parallel, in only a three to four degree of outward rotation, so that the hip joints, knees, and ankles can be properly aligned.

Always stand with your weight evenly distributed on both legs, unless you are able to place one foot up on a stool or a foot rest. Keep your knees slightly flexed. Feel your spine lengthening and your tailbone dropping to the floor like a kangaroo's tail. Feel the energy of your spine going up to the sky rather than dropping down and giving in to gravity.

Prolonged standing is always a strain and should be avoided whenever possible. If you are required to stand for long periods of time, do the following: Bend your knees and slightly round your spine; raise your knee to your chest or shift your weight from one foot to the other. Move as often as you can to prevent compression in any point of the body for a prolonged period of time.

SLEEPING

Myth: Sleeping on your back is recommended to prevent swayback.

Correction: Sleeping on the back is restful and correct only when the knees are properly supported.

Lying on your back with your knees bent and supported with a couple of pillows is the least stressful because it allows the lower back to lengthen out. Another good position is to lie on your side with both knees bent and one knee crossed over and slightly higher than the other. When sleeping on your side, use a pillow to maintain the position of your head in alignment with your trunk.

Sleeping prone (face down) is usually not recommended for people with lower back problems. The prone sleeping position is the most stressful to the lower back, because it accentuates the swayback position. However, this can be done if you do the following—bend one knee up toward your upper body, or place a pillow under your pelvis or chest (depending on where the back pain is located).

Getting out of Bed

Never sit bolt upright. After a relaxing night's sleep your muscles have released and lengthened out. To sit up quickly requires a muscular contraction, which can be very stressful to the back after being relaxed.

The proper way to get out of bed is to bend your knees slightly, roll over onto your side, and then to push your body up with your hands as you gently lower your feet to the floor. Keeping your lower spine tucked under and knees slightly bent, push up with your arms until you can raise up to vertical with your thighs. Do this every time you come up to a sitting position after sleeping, exercising, or getting off the doctor's examination table.

BENDING AND LIFTING

> *Myth:* Proper lifting techniques are only necessary when lifting heavy loads.
>
> *Correction:* Picking up *any* kind of load must be performed with the knees bent so that the legs share in the workload to avoid putting stress on the lower back.

If you have to move an object, realistically assess whether or not you can move it by yourself. If there is any doubt, ask for help. If there is no one to help you, don't move the object.

If you are going to pick up a heavy object, bend your knees and squat down in front of the object and lift it above your waist and close to your body. To stand up, just straighten your knees into the upright position. Never bend the torso forward without bending the knees and bending in the hip joints.

If you are going to lift and carry a heavy object on your back, such as a backpack, place your back to the object, bend your knees, and drop your lower spine as you hoist it onto your back. Exhale as you stretch up to vertical.

If you must carry a heavy shoulder bag, don't let it just hang from one shoulder. Place the strap over your head and across your body so that you can balance the weight from one shoulder to the opposite hip. Always try to keep yourself as balanced as possible. If you wear your bag or carry your briefcase across one shoulder when you go to work, try to remember to carry it on the opposite shoulder when you leave. If you're carrying a heavy package in one hand, try to shift it often to the other hand. If you use a backpack, don't drape it over one shoulder; position the straps properly over both shoulders to spread the weight evenly.

BACK PAIN PREVENTION—DO'S AND DON'TS

1. Do your exercise psoas stretches, back stretches, and abdominal strengtheners.
2. Whether standing, sitting, or lying in bed, learn to keep your head in line with your spine.

3. To prevent strain and pain in everyday activities, change from one task to another often to allow recovery and rest for the muscles before fatigue or spasm sets in.
4. Never lift or move heavy furniture. Let someone who knows the principles of leverage do it.
5. Never carry anything heavier than you can manage with ease.
6. Never bend from the waist. Bend the knees and the hip joints.
7. Never lift a heavy object higher than your waist.
8. Avoid carrying unbalanced loads; hold heavy objects close to your body.
9. Avoid high heels. Wear shoes with moderate heels, and change your heel height often to avoid putting too much stress on one muscle group.
10. Buy a rocking chair. Rocking rests the back by changing the muscle groups used.

A FINAL CHECKLIST

1. Just as food must be taken day by day for constant refreshment, so must physical exertion be a constant in the attainment and maintenance of a healthy body. Are you doing your exercises on a consistent basis?
2. Are you aware of postural malfunctioning? Are you able to visualize the changes you want to make?
3. Are you getting enough sleep? Are you sleeping on a good, hard mattress? Are you using pillow support where necessary?
4. Are you aware of the things that cause undue tension during your day? Are you aware of the stresses that can precipitate a lower-back muscle spasm?
5. Are you taking short breaks to relieve any tension accumulating in your back—at work, at the checkout counter, in your car, and so on?
6. Are you wearing good, supportive shoes that absorb impact and cushion your steps? Have you been alternating your low-heeled shoes with flats to reduce muscle strain?

Especially for Dancers

THE DANCER'S POSTURE

Posture and dance training are intimately connected. Graceful and poised, a dancer stands out in a crowd. Posture is any momentary stationary attitude the body assumes. Every physical activity is really a series of attitudes, which differ in sports, work habits and everyday movements. All movements must be mechanically efficient or they will subject the body to strain. Good posture is dynamic, not static, and takes less muscular effort to maintain than poor posture. Poor posture prevents the body from functioning properly, because the skeletal structure is out of alignment, and causes mechanical readjustment resulting in muscular effort and strain. The main contributing factors in chronic strain of the lower back are poor muscular control and poor body mechanics. Any departure from the balanced posture will strain muscles and ligaments and cause undue friction in joints.

THE DANCER'S BODY

Through proper training over a long period of time, dancers develop bodies that can withstand many physical stresses. Well-conditioned dancers will have stronger bones, ligaments and muscles than the more sedentary, non-dancers, and as a result will more easily adjust to torques and shock imposed by a particular dance form. However, even highly conditioned and skilled dancers may be predisposed to injury by adverse mechanical forces, such as abnormal angles of muscle pull, misalignment of body parts, a sudden forceful twist, or a breakdown in the normal synergy of a muscle or muscle group. Dancers often injure themselves as a result of taking improper or unnatural postures. They often attempt movements that are either beyond their particular capabilities or are inappropriate to their particular body build. Because dance is the epitome of motor control and physical endurance, inability to effectively perform over a long period of time with good body mechanics eventually leads dancers to sustain an acute or chronic injury.

Just as some individuals inherit organic susceptibilities to various diseases such as heart disease or hypertension, individuals inherit peculiarities in body structure that may or may not decrease their ability to withstand physical stresses. Often dancers' awareness of a potential physical weakness can be dealt with positively by employing better conditioning methods and avoiding activities that may aggravate the problem or prolong it.

THE CENTER OF STRENGTH

When dancers are "placed," the muscles of the torso have been so trained and developed that the physical demands of dancing can be handled with adequate muscular control without loss of poise or presence. The true strength of dancers lies in the muscles of their trunk. Flexibility of the spine and strong abdominal muscles give the feeling of "lightness" to dancers when they leap or land after a jump. The spinal column is a structure of stability and adaptation; an instrument of great precision and yet of robust durability.

Only a flexible back can be a strong back; flexibility of the spinal column can be gained through exercises that release and yet control the vertebral muscles. Rigidity in the torso is harmful to the moving body.

The traditional ballet barre is excellent training for strength and control necessary for the muscles of the torso. However, flexibility of the spine and back is essential for the dancer's technical prowess. Only when a muscle is able to contract and release in its full range of motion is strength possible.

The very nature of their intense activity renders dancers prone to injury and the torso is an area of particular vulnerability. For example, arching and overextension of the spine in an arabesque can occur if a male dancer has not been instructed in the correct method of lifting a female dancer.

OVERUSE SYNDROME

Dance, like any other strenuous, repetitious activity, can provide performers with an outstanding opportunity to develop well-conditioned bodies. However, if dance movements are improperly performed, or if movements are attempted that are beyond a dancer's skill level, the result may be a breakdown of supporting muscle and ligmentous structures followed by serious postural deviations or injury.

ARABESQUE

A "bad back" and a good *arabesque* don't mix. Hyperextending or arching the lower back can lead to low back problems. The action of raising the leg to the rear and perpendicular to the upper back causes tremendous shortening and tightening of the muscles of the lower back. In many cases, the muscles of the lower back are already short and tight, and the *arabesque* just forces muscles to be even tighter. The answer is not to force all the movement at the bottom of the spine, but to spread the extension throughout all the joints of the spine and, of course, prepare the body for this activity by stretching the muscles of the low back before performing this movement.

GRAND BATTEMENT

The action of the psoas muscle will bring the leg up to the torso as in *grand battement* or passè, or it will bring the torso to the legs, as in a full sit-up.

The *grand battement* is a movement that places a great deal of strain on the hip joint. To avoid unnecessary stress, the performer must hold the torso erect and keep the supporting leg straight at all times, with the pelvis and torso in as correct alignment as possible. Incorrect technique can lead to low back pain and hip problems. And, the repetition of this movement overly tightens the iliopsoas muscle, so stretching of the psoas is essential.

DOUBLE LEG LIFTS AND SIT-UPS

Some modern dance or jazz techniques and choreography may require a movement like a straight leg sit-up or a double leg lift from the floor. These movements must be avoided, because each places great strain on the lower back that can ultimately lead to chronic back problems. In both cases the iliopsoas is contracted, accentuating the lumbar curve of the lower back, and forced to tighten even more to complete the movement. As stated previously, the psoas muscle will bring the torso to the legs. When a person performs a full sit-up to the vertical position, the abdominal muscles are used in approximately thirty degrees of that activity, with the remainder of the work being done by the psoas group. Since the problem of an overly-tightened psoas is usually the case, we do not need to tighten it any further. There are modifications of these movements that can prevent lower back strain, such as a single leg lift so that the opposite foot can press on the floor to provide stability for the lower back. Or an abdominal curl can be done with the knees bent, with a roll to the side, so that the performer is using momentum and other muscles to assist in coming up to vertical.

SPINAL DEVIATIONS

Fortunately, serious disabling injuries of the back are unusual in a dancer who has a normal spine. However, certain defects of the spine may go unnoticed until a dancer is challenged with a heavy schedule of classes and rehearsals.

One such defect, called spondylolysis, is found in approximately five percent of the population, and dancers have a higher incidence of this condition than the general population. Spondylolysis is a crack in the posterior segment of a vetebral body, which can result in spondylolisthesis, a slippage of the vertebral body, forward on the vertebra below it. Spondylolysis, often can be asymptomatic throughout life. However, if this defect is present, numerous small stress fractures can occur to the vertebra progressing to slippage, because of the dancer's continual movement of the spine. This condition may be a contraindication for a dancer's acceptance into a company or school. Operative fusion of the joint may be a necessary treatment in severe cases, but symptoms may abate with rest and proper conservative treatment. Often the severity of the resulting back pain is not related to the slippage, but rather to the amount of muscle spasm from the instability of the vertebra and to the impingement of the disk on the spinal nerves.

Most dancers, fortunately do not have to contend with disk disease and spondylolisthesis, but they may have problems with muscle strains and sprains. Poor posture, bad placement and attempting to exceed basic anatomical limitations may all lead to back injury. Male dancers suffer more back strains, because of the lifting they do. In partnering, males should avoid excessive arching of the lower spine, and should strengthen the abdominal muscles and the muscles of the shoulders and arms as a preventive measure.

Because the back has a more natural inclination for muscle spasm rather than strain, ice massage combined with easy, slow stretching can relieve most symptoms. Any back pain that does not respond to a couple of days of reduced activity combined with gentle stretching exercises and the application of ice or moist heat should be sufficient reason to contact a health professional or physician.

SLIPPED DISKS

Although it is not my intention to go into great detail on the more serious pathological condition of "slipped disks," I will make mention of it since it can occur in the dancer's routine. A dancer can have a disk that has extruded or slipped out of place from between the vertebrae and then spontaneously go back into place. The muscles of the spine will go into spasm at the onset of pain caused by the disk displacement. This is an attempt to "splint" and protect the back against incautious, painful movement. Thus, begins the "vicious cycle." The pain causes the muscle to spasm and tighten to prevent further movement from injuring the area. However, because the muscle is in spasm, the afflicted person is forced to move in a stiff and timid fashion, which in and of itself becomes painful. This cycle can be broken by stretching exercises to break down the adhesion of muscle fibers caused by the spasm. If stretching exercise does not relieve the spasm, consult your regular physician before going elsewhere for spinal manipulation. It is extremely important that "slipped disks" and spondylolisthesis not be manipulated. What is therapeutic in one instance can be disastrous in another. When a disk "slips," future trouble is eliminated if it is returned to its original position as soon as possible. This should be followed by a series of stretching exercises for the back and psoas, and strengtheners for the abdominals.

STRESS AND THE DANCER

When considering injuries associated with psychogenic factors, one must consider muscular tension as a major cause in the dance field. Tension is defined as increased muscular contraction as a result of some emotional state or muscular work. Nervous tension is a syndrome that is characteristic of our times. An over-anxious dancer can have an extremely high level of unnecessary muscular tension. The person who is anxious outwardly may be less flexible and less able to smoothly coordinate muscles.

The tense dancer is extemely susceptible to injury. The ability to eliminate muscular tension by consciously "letting go" is very important to all dancers. Dancers who can relax at will can increase their mental and physical efficiency.

Although anxiety must be controlled when the dancer is engaged in an activity over a long period of time, pre-performance tension is a normal part of getting prepared for a first-rate performance. Once onstage, the professional soon forgets the fear and performs with a maximal expenditure of energy. A person's mental and emotional characteristics have a great deal to do with his or her ability to relax. Through breathing and visualization, a dancer can consciously "let go" of the tension in the muscles.

The best natural sedative and most effective tension pacifier is slow, deep breathing. You can condition yourself to associate your deep breathing with a conscious "letting go" as you exhale. The moment a dancer feels the tension begin to mount, he/she should take a deep breath and keep the breathing slow and long. Focusing attention on deep breathing will allow the muscles to release and "let go." Try to remember that a few deep breaths taken slowly and easily will always help you calm down and prepare you for a poised, efficient performance.

Dancers in a touring company sleep in a variety of beds, some hard, some soft, some sagging. A bed that sags is the worst and should be supported by a sheet of plywood. Since that solution would be difficult on tour, the backache sufferer can often obtain relief by lying supine on the floor with a folded towel supporting the low back curve and pillows to support bent knees. And don't forget to STRETCH! STRETCH! STRETCH!

PREPARING THE BODY TO PREVENT INJURY

One of the most important factors in dance training is the preparation of the body to endure the rigors of physical stress. Every dancer must have an appropriate degree of strength, muscular and cardiovascular endurance, and flexibility.

Strength is one of the dancer's most important concerns. Strength is defined as the capacity of the individual to exert a muscle contraction or force against a resistance. When muscles are exercised regularly certain physiological changes occur, including muscle size.

Because strength, in general, allows the dancer to move freely and handle the body efficiently, it also plays an extremely important role in the prevention of injury. However, for strength to be more effective, it must be properly balanced between the agonist and antagonist muscles. Therefore, a dancer concerned with injury prevention should be concerned with all-around muscle development, avoiding overdeveloping the strength of specific muscle groups.

Stamina—or muscle endurance and cardiovascular endurance—is the staying power of the body in a given activity or activities. Because dancing can be one of the most grueling endeavors, the efficient use of the heart, lungs and circulatory system is vital. The efficiency of the cardiovascular system is inseparable from the other components of the dancer's physical fitness. The body cannot be used effectively as a tool for creative expression without all physical fitness factors being at the highest level possible.

Flexibility—the ability to move the joints through full range of motion—is the most important physiological factor in the prevention of dance injuries. The human body varies greatly in its ability to engage in a broad spectrum of movement. There can be many causes for an increase or decrease in joint flexibility—physiological, anatomical or even emotional.

When considering flexibility, one must be reminded how posture and daily habit patterns can affect the joints and alter the range of motion. Or a joint that is heavily bound by ligaments may be more restricted than a loosely supported joint. Bulky muscles and tight, unyielding tendons can also restrict the range of motion. Although most restricted movements of joints are of an anatomical or physiological origin, a person's mental and emotional characteristics have a great deal to do with the ability to relax. The tense individual who appears restricted and withdrawn because of painful emotions often reflects these feelings in a rigid and unyielding body.

To achieve a lithe and flexible body one must do stretching exercises. However, at this point I would like to mention the ineffective and "bad" stretching that has often been taught to dance students. The "bad" stretching that I am referring to is ballistic stretching, or more accurately "ballistic bouncing." Ballistic bouncing or stretching is a pulsating movement to supposedly increase the length of a particular muscle or muscle group. Uncontrolled ballistic bouncing is dangerous because it can adversely affect supporting ligaments and may result in muscle spasm by causing a reflexive contraction of the muscle rather than the desired release and stretch. Ballistic movements stimulate the "stretch reflex," which aggravates muscle tissue and possibly causes minor tearing of the muscle tissue and, therefore, causes it to spasm.

Stretching exercises are most effective when executed slowly and deliberately rather than with bouncing or jerking movements. When performing a stretching exercise, you place yourself in the desired position of the stretch, relax and gradually try to release a little further into it thereby achieving a greater stretch. To increase the lengthening phase, *exhale* to allow the stretched muscle to release fully.

It is not my intention to present an extensive discussion of individual endurance, strength and flexibility exercises that a dancer might perform, but to present specific exercises selected for their ability to increase flexibility of the lower back, hip and groin areas to prevent specific injuries.

Workout Sequence #5

1. *Relaxing Adductor Stretch*
2. *Rock and Stretch*
3. *Adductor Stretch with Supporting Leg Bent and with Standing Leg Long*
4. *Vertical Adductor Stretch and Adductor Stretch Tilted Forward*
5. *Second Position Stretch with Pelvis Support*
6. *Second Position with Head Support*
7. *Inverted Second Position*
8. *Long Sit on Pillows*
9. *Inverted Back Stretch*
10. *Thoracic Lift*
11. *Inverted Legs on Chair*

1. *Relaxing Adductor Stretch*

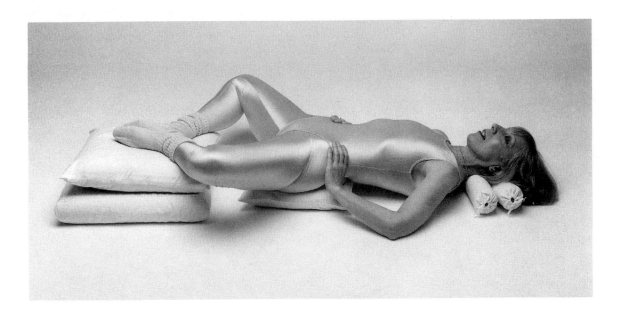

POSITION/ACTIVITY: Lie supine with your pelvis supported on a pillow, your head supported by a pillow, and your feet resting on pillow support.

IMAGE: Visualize your thighs spiraling outward from the hip joint down to the knees.

DURATION: Two minutes.

2. Rock and Stretch

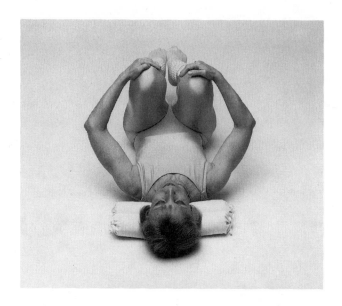

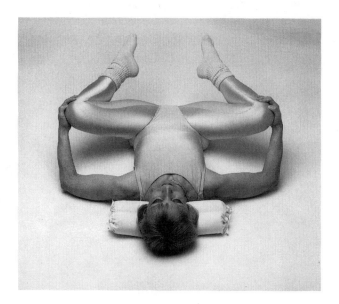

POSITION: Lie supine, with your knees raised to your chest, placing hands
on top of knees.

ACTIVITY 1:   Circle your thighs away from the center line of the torso.

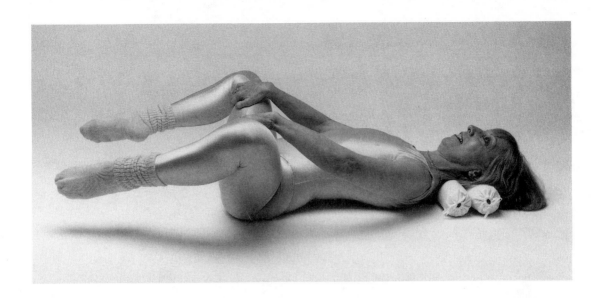

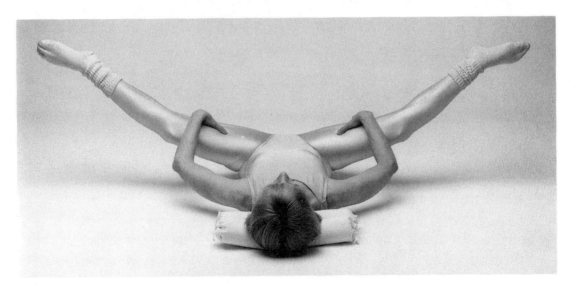

ACTIVITY 2:	Place your hands inside the thighs and gently rock pelvis forward and back.
ACTIVITY 3:	Slowly extend legs out to the side, but never fully straighten the knees.
IMAGE:	Visualize the energy of the thighs as it spirals out from your center all the way through your toes.
DURATION:	Two minutes.

Especially for Dancers **251**

3. Adductor Stretch with Supporting Leg Bent and with Standing Leg Long

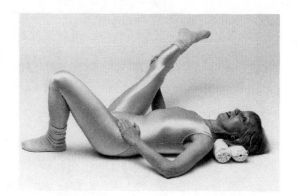

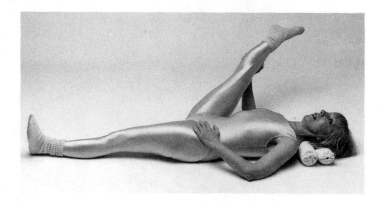

POSITION 1:	Lie supine, with your left knee bent and foot flat on the floor.
ACTIVITY:	Extend your right leg out to the side and keep your left hip bone on the floor.
IMAGE:	Visualize your lower back and pelvis widening and expanding sideways as you visualize your right leg spiraling away from your center.
DURATION:	One minute.
POSITION 2:	Lie supine, with your left leg lengthened down along the floor.
ACTIVITY:	Extend your right leg out to the side and keep your left hip bone on the floor.
IMAGE:	Visualize the length of your supporting left side as you visualize your right leg spiralling out away from your center.
DURATION:	One minute.

4. *Vertical Adductor Stretch and Adductor Stretch Tilted Forward*

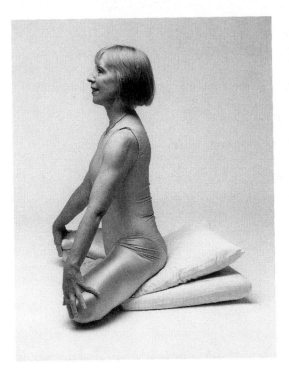 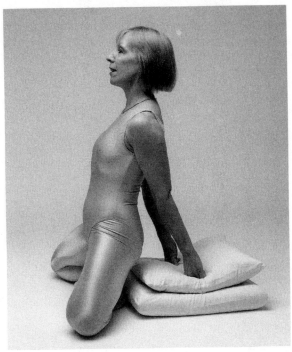

POSITION/ACTIVITY 1:	Sit on firm pillows with your knees bent and dropped sideways down to the floor.
IMAGE:	Feel the support from your pelvis traveling up the spine and out through the top of your head, as you visualize your thighs spiraling outward from the hip joint to the knees.
DURATION:	Thirty seconds.
POSITION/ACTIVITY 2:	Place your hands on the pillow behind you and raise your buttocks off the pillow.
IMAGE:	Feel the length of your spine travelling upwards, as you visualize your thighs spiralling outward from the hip joints to the knees.
DURATION:	Thirty seconds.

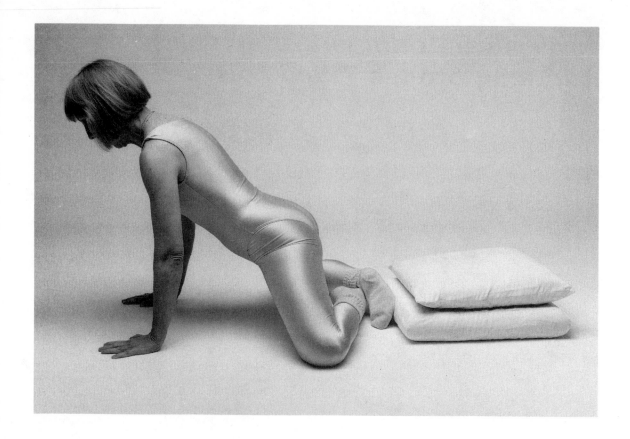

POSITION/ACTIVITY 3:	Transfer your weight from the hands behind you, to the hands in front of you.
IMAGE:	Visualize your pelvis dropping forward to the floor and your thighs rotating outward from your center.
DURATION:	Thirty seconds.

5. *Second Position Stretch with Pelvis Support*

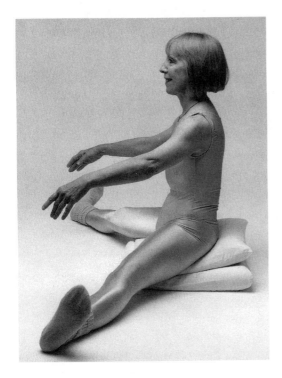
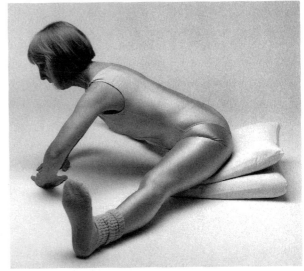

POSITION:	Sit on firm pillows, with your legs opened wide and your pelvis tilted back.
ACTIVITY:	Sit upright on your "sitz-bones" and bring your arms forward.
IMAGE:	Visualize the length of your spine from your tailbone to the top of your head and your thighs rotating outward from the hip joints all the way down through your feet.
DURATION:	Two minutes.

6. *Second Position with Head Support*

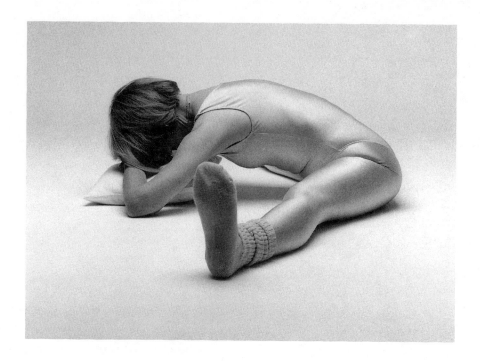

POSITION: Sit, with your legs opened wide.

ACTIVITY: Drop your head and hands on a pillow and allow your back to
                   relax.

IMAGE: Visualize the energy of your thighs spiraling outward from your
                   hip joints all the way through your feet.

DURATION: Two minutes.

7. *Inverted Second Position*

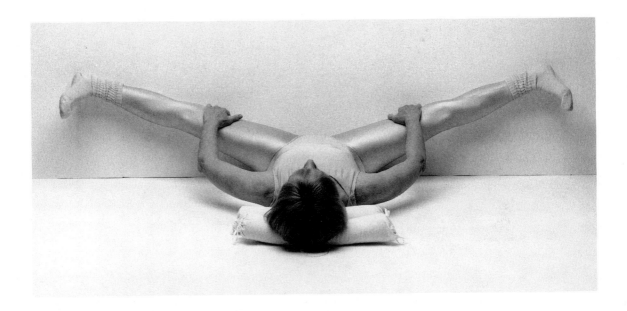

POSITION: Lie supine, with your legs extended to the ceiling and your heels resting against the wall.

ACTIVITY: Inhale, then exhale as you allow your legs to relax and open wide to your sides.

IMAGE: Imagine that the energy of your thighs is rotating and spiraling out away from your center.

DURATION: Two minutes.

8. *Long Sit on Pillows*

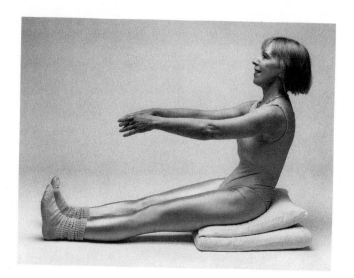

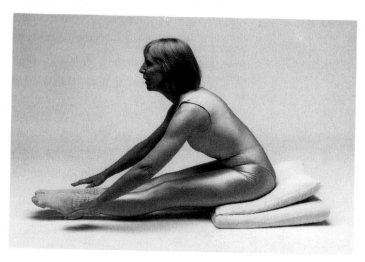

POSITION:	Sit on firm pillows, with your legs extended forward.
ACTIVITY:	Tilt your pelvis backwards and then tilt your pelvis forward as you reach your hands toward your feet.
IMAGE:	Imagine that the energy from your center radiates from the pelvis all the way up the spine and from lower spine down through the legs.
DURATION:	Two minutes.

9. *Inverted Back Stretch*

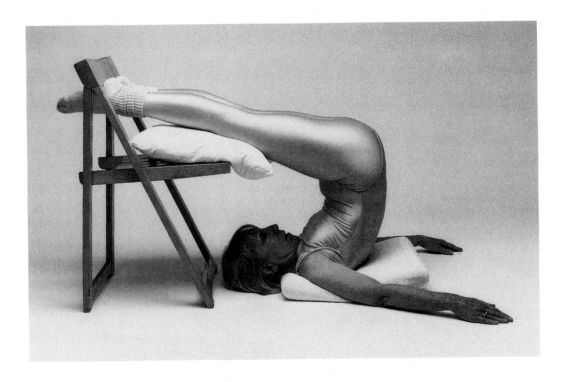

POSITION:	Lie supine, with your legs raised over head and resting on a chair.
ACTIVITY:	Inhale, and then exhale as you relax and release into the stretch.
IMAGE:	Imagine that your breath opens and releases all the tight spots along your spine, head, neck and shoulders.
DURATION:	Two minutes.

10. *Thoracic Lift*

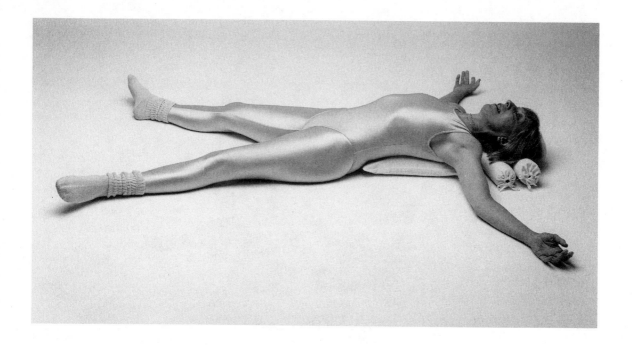

POSITION:	Lie supine, with a firm pillow to support your rib-cage and upper back.
ACTIVITY:	Inhale, and then exhale.
IMAGE:	Imagine that you are a five-pointed star with energy radiating from your center.
DURATION:	Two minutes.

11. *Inverted Legs on Chair*

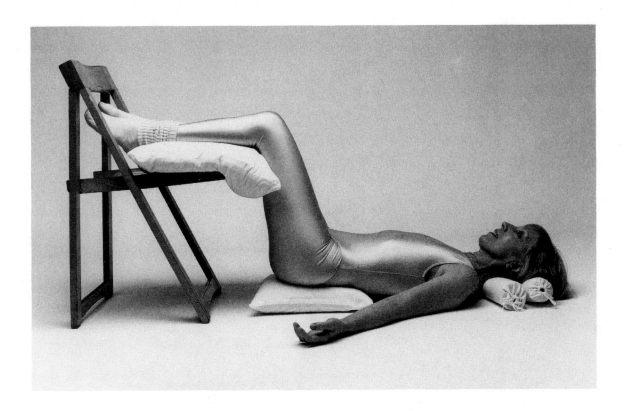

POSITION:	Lie supine, with your knees bent and your legs resting on a chair.
ACTIVITY:	Inhale, and then exhale.
IMAGE:	Imagine that you feel the weight of the legs pouring back down to the pelvis, and then visualize the length of your spine from the tail-bone all the way to the top of the head.
DURATION:	Two minutes.

Glossary

Aerobic exercise

Physical activity that uses the large muscle groups and can be performed steadily and consistently for a long period of time. Working aerobically increases an individual's cardiovascular strength, muscular endurance, metabolic rate, and ability to burn fat as fuel. (Fat cannot be metabolized without oxygen.)

Alignment position

Proper mechanical balance, achieved when the arrangement of the skeletal structure is such that a stable equilibrium is maintained in the upright position without outside help. The body is in proper alignment when the feet are on the floor with the toes parallel and facing forward, in line with the ankle joint, knee joint, and hip joint, and the weight is distributed equally and as close as possible to the central line of gravity.

Anaerobic exercise

Physical activity of high intensity that can only be performed for a short duration because it is done without oxygen as fuel. Instead, anaerobic metabolism uses the muscle stores of carbohydrate (glycogen) for energy. Sprinting is an example of anaerobic exercise.

Concave

Describing the inside line of a curve.

Convex

Describing the outside line of a curve.

Cool-down period

The period following exercise when the body's temperature and heart rate return to normal resting levels.

Exhalation

The forceful expulsion of air from the lungs.

Flex   The bent position of a joint, placed with control.

Glucose   Carbohydrate breakdown resulting in blood sugar level for energy source.

Glycogen   Glucose as it is stored in the muscles or liver.

Iliopsoas   Actually a composite of two muscles, the psoas major and the iliacus. The psoas major has its origin just below the twelfth thoracic vertebra attaching to the five lumbar vertebrae proceeding diagonally through the abdominal cavity, serving with shelflike function for some of the internal organs, and inserting to the inner side of the thigh bone. The iliacus is a flat triangular muscle that extends from the inner border of the hipbone to the inner side of the thighbone.

Inhalation   Taking breath in until the lungs are full.

Kinesthetic   Describing the sensation of movement in the muscles, tendons, and joints.

Lumbar lordosis   Swayback.

Neuromuscular patterning   The method whereby, on impulse from the central nervous system, electrochemical energy is transformed into kinetic energy, which then sets the muscles into motion.

Prone   Lying face down.

Supine   Lying on the back, face upward.

Suggested Reading

Chapter 1

Birnbaum, M.D., Jacob S. *The Musculoskeletal Manual*. New York: Academic Press, 1982.

Johnson, Don. *The Protean Body*. New York: Harper Colophon Books, 1977.

Michele, Arthur A. *Iliopsoas*. Springfield, Illinois: Charles C. Thomas, 1962.

Michele, Arthur A. *Orthotherapy*. New York: M. Evans & Co., 1971.

Chapter 2

Barlow, Wilfred. *The Alexander Technique*. New York: Alfred A. Knopf, 1973.

Benson, M.D., Herbert. *The Relaxation Response*. New York: Avon Books, 1975.

Feldenkrais, Moshe. *Awareness Through Movement*. New York: Harper & Row, 1972.

Sweigard, Lulu E. *Human Movement Potential: Its Ideokinetic Facilitation*. New York: Harper & Row, 1974.

Todd, Mabel Ellsworth. *The Thinking Body*. New York: Dance Horizons, 1937.

Todd, Mabel Ellsworth. *The Hidden You*. New York: Exposition Press, 1953.

Chapter 5

Bailey, Covert. *Fit or Fat*. Boston: Houghton Mifflin Co., 1977.

Bennett, M.D., William, and Joel Gurin. *The Dieter's Dilemma*. New York: Basic Books, 1982.

Brody, Jane. *Jane Brody's Good Food Book*. New York: Ballantine Books, 1979.

Brody, Jane. *Jane Brody's Nutrition Book*. New York: W. W. Norton & Co., 1981.

Colbin, Annemarie. *Food and Healing*. New York: Ballantine Books, 1986.

Malkin, Mort. *Walking: The Pleasure Exercise*. Emmaus, Pennsylvania: Rodale Press, 1986.

McGee, Harold. *On Food and Cooking*. New York: Scribners, 1984.

Sweetgall, Robert. *Fitness Walking*. New York: Perigree Books, 1986.

Chapter 6

Brewer, Gail Sforza. *Nine Months, Nine Lessons*. New York: Simon & Schuster, 1983.

Nobel, R.P.T., Elizabeth. *Essential Exercises for the Childbearing Year*. Boston: Houghton Mifflin Co., 1982.

Chapter 7

Adams, R. D. *Diseases of Muscle*, 3rd ed. Hagerstown, Maryland: Harper, 1975.

Friedmann, M.D., Lawrence W., and Lawrence Galton. *Freedom from Backaches*. New York: Pocket Books, 1973.

Klein, Arthur C., and Dava Sobel. *Backache Relief*. New York: New American Library, 1986.

Levine, M.D., David B. *The Painful Low Back*. New York: PW Communications, 1979.

White, III, M.D., Augustus A. *Your Aching Back, A Doctor's Guide to Relief*. New York: Bantam Books, 1983.

Index